I0414730

A
RETROSPECTIVE
REVIEW
of Patient Satisfaction Scores and the Relationship to
PATIENT CENTERED
MEDICAL HOME
Implementation

By

Jacquelene S. Hamer-McGhee, DNP, MSA, RN

Jacquelene S. Hamer-McGhee, DNP, MSA, RN

Abstract

The U.S. Department of Health and Human Services (HHS) and the Affordable Care Act (ACA) place patients in the center of all health care decisions and empower them with choices to drive health care delivery (U.S. Department of Health and Human Services, 2014). Since the enactment of the ACA, health care organizations have been under increased pressure to improve metrics of patient satisfaction scores, cost base, and health care outcomes (Glenn, 2012). To assist health care leaders with improving metrics, reemphasis is placed on implementing an enhanced model of primary care such as the Patient Centered Medical Home (PCMH). Health care administrators and leaders tend to overlook how implementing PCMH affects patients' satisfaction scores despite the evidence to support improving quality in the primary health care environments. A non-experimental quantitative analysis approach was used to guide the project in addition to a foundational theoretical framework derived from Donabedian's framework for health care quality. The results of the project supported the rejection of the null hypothesis, there is a relationship between the overall CAHPS scores and the number of PCMH facilities (p-value is less than 0.001) by regions in the United States for years 2012 and 2013. A statistically significant difference also existed in the mean scores between year and satisfaction and between region and PCMH total. The number of PCMH facilities for the year and region totals had p-values of 0.051 and <0.001, respectively. The p-value of 0.051 was not significant. There was not a statistical significance in the mean scores between the PCMH total and year. There was a statistical significance for PCMH and region.

Keywords: Patient Satisfaction, Patient-Centered Care, Team-based Care

Jacquelene S. Hamer-McGhee, DNP, MSA, RN

Acknowledgments

There were many wonderful people for whom I am truly grateful to have in my life and who have helped to pull me through this pruning and learning process, but all honor and glory goes to God! I give many thanks to Dr. Judy Burckhardt, my committee chair for her flexibility and patience with the submission of my work and for truly being encouraging and concerned; To Dr. Eddie Beard and Dr. Heidi Landry, my committee members for their candid, yet gentle approach to mentoring; To Dr. Olivia Scott for her unconditional friendship and professional guidance.

To my husband Cliff who is my biggest "DNP" cheerleader. He kept me focused, cared for me, and even woke up in the early morning hours, when I could no longer see, to proofread my papers. To my mother Trudy who has instilled in me to never give up. To my sister Kim, for her unconditional support; To Wanda, for her sponsorship, her weekly mental health checks, and her solution for everything… the spa; To my sisters in Christ from Bible Study Fellowship, for their prayers and bonding; and to my daughters, Brandi, Jessica, and Ariel for whom I must set the example.

Jacquelene S. Hamer-McGhee, DNP, MSA, RN

Contents

Jacquelene S. Hamer-McGhee, DNP, MSA, RN

CHAPTER 1
Introduction

The U.S. Department of Health and Human Services (HHS) and the Affordable Care Act (ACA) place patients in the center of all health care decisions and empower them with choices to drive the delivery of their health care (U.S. Department of Health and Human Services, 2014). Since the health care reform bill passed on March 21, 2010, health care organizations have been under increased pressure to improve metrics of patient satisfaction scores, cost base, and health care outcomes (Glenn, 2012). To assist health care leaders, improve the metrics, emphasis is placed on implementing an enhanced model of primary care. For the purpose of this project, the investigator examined the Patient Centered Medical Home (PCMH) model. The Agency for Health and Research Quality (AHRQ) defines PCMH as: "A model of care for delivering primary care that is patient-centered, comprehensive, team-based, and coordinated among all health care providers. Patient Centered Medical Homes also allow better access to care and are continuously improved through a systems-based approach to quality and safety" (AHRQ, 2013, p. 1). The tenants of PCMH consist of access to care, communication between patient and provider, helpful and courteous staff, and provider ratings (CAHPS, 2011). Prior to 2010, little emphasis was placed on implementing PCMH. Passage of the Health care Reform bill required facilities to implement enhanced models of care (PCMH).

Rozenblum et al. (2013) identified a gap in the knowledge base that suggests leaders and health care providers fail to have a structured plan in place to improve patients' satisfaction. The lack of patient involvement in the comprehensive decision-making process leads to poor patient satisfaction scores. According to Consumer of Health Assessment of Providers and Systems (CAHPS, 2011), patients' satisfaction scores are measured by four composites: access to care, communication, helpful staff, and provider scoring. CAHPS is a public program initiative supported by AHRQ to develop standardized surveys of patients' experiences. This project strived to examine if the implementation of a PCMH model of care influenced patients' experiences reported in the form of patients' satisfaction scores. The investigator examined the effects by determining if there is a relationship between patients' satisfaction scores and PCMH implemented facilities in four regions of the U.S.

Problem Statement

Health care administrators and leaders tend to overlook how implementing PCMH affects patients' satisfaction scores despite the evidence to support improving quality in the primary health care environments. According to Rozenblum et al., (2013) and Becker (2013), health care providers and administrators also struggle to acknowledge that poor customer service, lack of patient-centered care, and the lack of patient engagement are the most likely causes of poor patients' satisfaction scores.

A Patient-Centered Medical Home is a model that focuses on patient-centered care and teamwork. Furlow (2014) hypothesized that implementation of the PCMH model would address both patients' satisfaction scores and provide patient-centered care. A Study by Cooley, MacAllister, Sherrieb, and Kuhlthau (2009) suggested that interventions implemented using PCMH concepts helped improve patients' satisfaction scores. Oldenburg, Chase, Christensen, and Trittle (2013) found that low patients' satisfaction scores appear to have a negative effect on health care outcomes and the entire health care system's bottom line.

Jacquelene S. Hamer-McGhee, DNP, MSA, RN

Background

The face of health care has rapidly changed since the IOM published, *Crossing the Quality Chasm* in 2001. From Carlstrom and Ekman's (2012) perspective, health care systems across the globe face challenges to meet the complexity of elevated health care costs and treatment needs for an increasing population of patients with chronic disorders. Past methods and strategies for maintaining a robust health care organization have slowly trickled away. Health care leaders are now expected to take what is left and function with new technology, innovation, and culture changes for today's consumers of care. To meet this challenge, realignment of health care systems' structure and outdated clinical processes must take effect in organizations to accommodate chronic care management as an essential health care goal of the PCMH model (Carlstrom & Ekman, 2012).

To start the process of changing outdated clinical processes and realignment of health care systems, patients were given a new bill of rights through the comprehensive health reform bill and the Patient Protection Affordable Care Act (PPACA), which was signed into law March 23, 2010 (Rozenblum et al., 2013). Since the passing of the comprehensive health reform bill and the PPACA in 2010, an increased urgency for improved primary care models, access to care and patient satisfaction initiatives exists. Even though the lack of patient engagement, low patient satisfaction scores, and poor access to care continued to elevate health care costs and produce unacceptable health care outcomes, hospital administrators, and health care providers continued to overlook the importance of a structured plan to improve customer service and patient satisfaction (Rozenblum et al., 2013).

Becker (2013) and Greene, Tuzzio, and Cherkin (2012) make good arguments for patient-centered care and patient satisfaction in that health care executives have not directed all aspects of their operational and clinical resources towards placing the patient in the center of health care delivery. Patient-centeredness and customer service are critical elements of a PCMH structure that health care leaders must embrace and understand to ensure this same message reaches those expected to deliver patient-centered care. The support and action of all health care professionals for patient-centered care is essential to maximize patient satisfaction, communication, clinical workflow processes, and resources that support the new structure throughout the organization (Tremblay et al., 2014).

Evidence of little to no patient-centered care or customer service is manifested in patients' frequent use of the emergency room because of the unavailability of same day appointments with assigned health care providers. Readmissions to the hospital in less than 30 days from date of discharge because of poor communication and lack of discharge instructions are also a result of poor patient-centered care. To address these issues, the Hospital Consumer Assessment of Healthcare Providers & Systems (HCAHPS) surveys were designed to report-patients' satisfaction scores and measures for in-patients. The measures reported for HCAHPS include: Nurse and physician communicaiton with the patient; patient receipt of timely care, pain control, explaination of medication; cleanliness of patient environment; noise control at night; and explaination of care provided (need citation)

For this project, the focus was on CAHPS surveys to measure patient satisfaction in the outpatient clinician and group practice environments. The HCAHPS and CAHPS surveys are related in that they both are designed to capture the patients' experience with health care and patient satisfaction. An additional similarity is that these examples of patient-centered care and health care access are believed to be directly linked to barriers of care and poor health care outcomes (IOM, 2012).

Jacquelene S. Hamer-McGhee, DNP, MSA, RN

Barriers that are believed to cause low patient satisfaction scores and poor access to care include: inadequate staffing for the clinic or in-patient care setting; staff burnout; non-availablity of appointments for scheduling; poor communication between providers and patients; poor language translation; lack of health insurance, low economic status; and disparities targeted at ethnicity, age, and gender (IOM, 2012) . According to Patel et al. (2013), the PCMH model proposes an innovative holistic approach to care that maximizes the communication, resources, and clinical processes needed to increase satisfaction scores and access to health care services. However, some researchers believe that the staffing requirements to implement and sustain this stucture have not been well defined and have caused leaders of health care organizations to hesitate to fully implement PCMH (Patel et al., 2013).

Purpose

The purpose of the project was to determine if there is a relationship between the overall CAHPS scores and the number of PCMH facilities by regions in the United States for calendar years 2012 and 2013. The researcher attempted to determine if there was a trend in the data. The intent of examining the relationship between PCMH implementation and patients' satisfaction scores was to provide health care executives with information they could use to make informed decisions about implementing an enhanced primary care concept based on patient experiences to increase patients' satisfaction and to support research that improves patients' satisfaction scores.

Significance of the Study

According to Centers for Medicare and Medicaid (CMS, 2014), patients' satisfaction and excellent customer service are significant for health care providers and administrators because patients' satisfaction is the driver for health care reimbursement and provider retention. Thirty percent of health care reimbursement is tied to how well patients rate their provider, which gives them an incentive to be more personable with their patients. Additionally, the Patient-Centered Primary Care Collaborative (PCPCC) suggested that PCMH is a model of health care delivery that is associated with lower health care costs and improved patients' satisfaction scores (PCPCC, 2007). The Patient-Centered Primary Care Collaborative also found that care delivered by primary care physicians in a PCMH model was consistently associated with better patient outcomes. As stated in an article by National Committee for Quality Assurance (NCQA, 2008):

The PCMH model of care was sought by practices to fortify the physician-patient relationship services by replacing episodic care with coordinated care and a long-term curative relationship. The PCMH model improved care through communication, access to care, staff courteousness, and provider ratings.

This project was selected because patients' satisfaction scores are not only an important and moral aspect of health care, they also have a direct effect on how patients respond to care (Brennan & Monson, 2014). The significance of this project was to determine if the implementation of PCMH is relational to overall patients' satisfaction scores. The results from the project indicated there was a correlation between the number of PCMH facilities and patients' satisfaction scores.

The Nature of the Project

The design for this project was a non-experimental quantitative analysis design utilizing secondary data to determine if there is a relationship between patients' satisfaction scores and the number of PCMH facilities that have been implemented across regions in the U.S. for years

2012 to 2013. The investigator extracted de-identified archived survey data from the online public CAHPS database. This project was conducted retrospectively by utilizing patient satisfaction survey results for health care facilities across the U.S. in four different regions (northern, southern, eastern, and western) over two consecutive years (2012 and 2013). Each region was examined to help determine if there were trends associated with the two variables. The result of the analysis was used to determine if a significant statistical correlation exists between patients' satisfaction scores and the number of PCMH facilities implemented across regions in the U.S.

The instrument used for extracting patient satisfaction data was the Consumer Assessment of Healthcare Providers and Systems (CAHPS)-Adult Visit Questionnaire (See Appendix B). The (CAHPS)-Adult Visit Questionnaire is a 37-item survey that captures patients' reports of their health care experiences. Four composites make up the body of the CAHPS survey: (a) timely appointments, care, and information; (b) how well providers communicate with patients; (c) helpful, courteous, and respectful office staff; and (d) patient ratings of their providers (needs citation). All CAHPS surveys are fielded by a third-party vendor that ensures assigned employees are properly trained according to the standards established by CAHPS before they are permitted to send the surveys out to eligible patients. Results for the CAHPS surveys are free and publicly available on the NCQA, PCPCC, CMS, and AHRQ websites.

Data analysis for this non-experimental quantitative study used Statistical Analysis Software (SAS) downloaded from a secure email link provided by the CAHPS database administrator upon request to use the dataset for research. Once the request to use the data was accepted, a signed acceptance of use agreement was forwarded to the CAHPS database administrator. Statistical Analysis Software (SAS) version 9.3 was used to organize, calculate, and analyze the research data.

A population of 50,000 patients over the age of 18 who were seen in a clinician or group practice over a one-year period comprised the total sample. A simple randomized sample of 25,000 patient responses in 2012 and 2013 across four regions (northern, southern, eastern, and western) was taken from the CAHPS database for analysis. Upon completion of this project, a determination was made as to whether there was a correlation between patients' satisfaction scores and the number of PCMH facilities across the U.S. in four different regions.

A simple randomized sample of 30 subjects for each region over two years (2012 and 2013) was extracted from the CAHPS database. The patient satisfaction data were examined for outliers, skewness, and kurtosis. Descriptive statistics were used to measure central tendency, measures of variability, and measures of relative standing throughout the project data. The hypothesis was assessed with a Pearson-*r* Correlation Coefficient instead of t-test.

Research Question

The research question guiding this project was based on four categories supporting PCMH and patients' satisfaction. This quantitative secondary analysis project measured data extracted from CG-CAHPS Adult Visit survey. The project focused on the four categories of patients' satisfaction surveys in relation to PCMH implemented health care facilities across four different regions of the U.S over a two-year period (2012 and 2013). The PCMH categories targeted include getting timely appointments, communication with patients; courteous hospital staff; and patients' rating of the provider (CAHPS, 2013) This capstone project answered the following research question:

What is the relationship between patients' satisfaction scores and the number of PCMH facilities across four regions in the U.S. for 2012 to 2013?

Jacquelene S. Hamer-McGhee, DNP, MSA, RN

Hypotheses

The null and alternative hypotheses were as follows:

H0: There is no relationship between patients' satisfaction scores and the number of PCMH health care facilities in different regions of the U.S. for 2012 to 2013.

H1: There is a relationship between patients' satisfaction scores and the number of PCMH health care facilities in different regions of the U.S. for 2012 to 2013.

Theoretical Framework

The Donabedian Quality Framework, first introduced by Dr. Avedis Donabedian in the 1966 seminal paper, "Evaluating the Quality of Medical Care", focused on evaluating processes in health care and how patients could benefit through their health outcomes. The Donabedian quality framework highlights relationship and change management concepts found in operational structures of care and process delivery (Spooner, Reese, & Konschak, 2012). Donabedian (needs date) defined this foundational framework of three dimensions to assess health care quality: structure, process, and outcomes.

This quality framework is part of many studies that include health care quality management, health information technology, and the development of quality measures that influence three dimensions of health care quality: structure of care, process of care, and health outcomes (Spooner et al., 2012).

The interactions and connection changes noted in Donabedian's framework among structure and clinical processes guided the capstone project to determine if there is a statistically significant difference between patients' satisfaction scores in PCMH- and NONPCMH-implemented health care facilities.

According to Morrison (2011), the definition for quality is approached from many perspectives that Donabedian observed as definitions of quality ordinarily reflected by the values and goals of the current medical care systems, as well as those of the larger society of which it is part.

Donabedian distinguished three aspects of care that are measured. The following three dimensions provide a deeper level of detail of Donabedian's quality framework as it applies to this project. It also highlights the framework's transformational qualities over time that makes it relevant for today's health care environment.

Structure

The architectural construct, correct staffing model, and health information technology must exist to fit the organizational primary care model of the Patient-Centered Medical Home (PCMH) model. Examples of the architectural construct include adequate space to ensure successful PCMH clinic workflow, proper information technology equipment (computers, software, documentation tools, and robust clinical dashboard for decision support) and medical equipment. Paustian et al. (2013) added health care production structure such as facilities management, logistics, pharmaceuticals, and other resources that augment the delivery of patient-centered health care to this dimension.

Process

The use of information technology integration with the electronic health record (EHR) and an organization's clinical and administrative processes for care delivery are examples of multi-dimensional processes that require clinical workflow analysis. This analysis would ensure that the clinical and business operational systems integrate with evidenced-based medical practices to drive improvement in clinical decision-making and patient satisfaction (Spooner et al., 2012).

Jacquelene S. Hamer-McGhee, DNP, MSA, RN

Other considerations for the process dimension are the extent to which professionals perform according to accepted standards, timeliness of care, appointment scheduling, available appointments, communication between patients and health care providers (secure messaging), and team-based care. Paustian et al. (2013) recommended examining whether the norms for Clinical Practice Guideline (CPG) procedures follow the medical practice recommendations to control underuse, misuse, or overuse of clinical tests, treatments, and diagnostic procedures.

Outcome

Outcome pertains to changes in the patient's condition following treatment and experience of care, such as patient satisfaction metrics, patient health care outcomes (such as improved diabetic control, asthma, and timely preventive screenings), and access to care. Paustian et al. (2013) highlighted the ultimate goals of reducing morbidity/mortality by improving the quality of life (QOL). Quality analysts identify problems by comparing outcomes achieved for patients with the outcomes projected for patients with the same disease. For example, high-quality care may be associated with a reduced frequency of relapses for patients with multiple sclerosis (MS) or uncontrolled diabetes, hypertension, and obesity.

This project ties into the Donabedian Theoretical Framework from a health care quality standpoint. The project highlights two specific quality aims from the IOM's *Crossing the Quality Chasm* report from 2001 (timely and patient-centered care). This project aimed to provide information to the research body of knowledge as well as health care leaders on the implementation of a process improvement initiative to help increase patient satisfaction scores. The PCMH model has multiple complex elements associated with the implementation, sustainment, and expected outcomes. The

Donabedian framework is one that can be used for its real-time capabilities to handle relationship and change management concepts that are commonly found in operational structures. The patient has the potential to gain benefits from coordinated quality care that promotes patient-centered care and patient satisfaction.

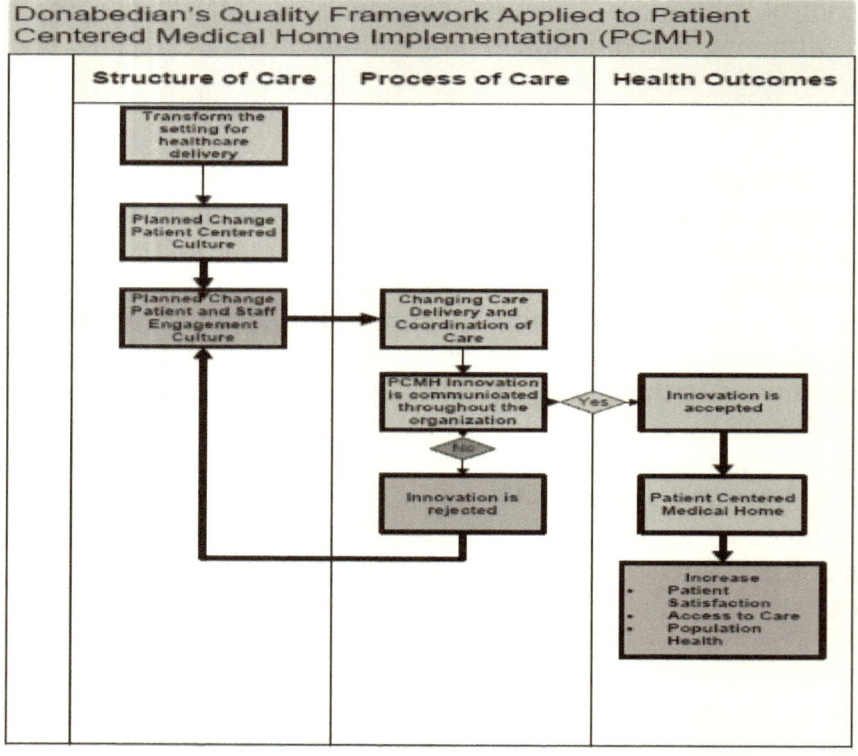

Figure 1. Attributes and Behaviors Needed to Provide Patient-Centered Care.
Data is adapted from Accountable Care: Bridging the HIT Divide (Spooner et al., 2012).

Jacquelene S. Hamer-McGhee, DNP, MSA, RN

Definitions

Care by design (CBD): A model of primary care focused on the concepts of holistic patient-centered care and a team-based approach. The structure of teams for CBD is different from PCMH and (Patient Alignment Care Team (PACT) in that CBD focuses more on process than structure.

Clinical practice guideline (CPG): The standards needed to judge the quality and reliability of existing clinical practices.

Consumer of Health Assessment of Providers and Systems (CAHPS): Supported by AHRQ, the CHAPS program is a public-private initiative to develop standardized surveys of patients' experiences. The survey covers ambulatory care and facility-level care with core and supplemental questions (access and wait times, patient-doctor communication, trust, continuity of care, coordination between primary care physicians and specialists, referrals, preventive care, experiences with office staff, and demographic characteristics). Health care organizations, public and private purchasers, consumers, and researchers use CAHPS results to assess patient-centered care, compare and report on performance, and improve quality of care. CAHPS survey results are obtained through AHRQ's national CAHPS Benchmarking Database, the National Committee for Quality Assurance, the HQA Hospital Compare website, and other pubic report cards.

Electronic health record (EHR): The Electronic Health Record is a software platform that systematically manages patient health information data for health care facilities.

Full time equivalent (FTE): A measurement used in business management to determine the level of time employees are required to work based on their position title and description (i.e., a full-time nurse practitioner would count for a full-time FTE of 0.75 hours).

Health Care Effectiveness Data and Information Set (HEDIS): A set of standardized measures designed by the

National Committee for Quality Assurance to evaluate the quality of health care and service provided by health plans and physicians.

Health information exchange (HIE): Provides the capability to move clinical data electronically between disparate health care information systems (clinical systems within a network) while maintaining the meaning of the information being exchanged. The goal of HIEs is to facilitate access and retrieval of clinical data to provide safer, timelier, efficient, effective, equitable, patient-centered care.

Institute of Medicine (IOM): A not-for-profit, non-governmental organization chartered in 1970 that provides national advice on issues related to biomedical science, medicine, and health. The organization serves as an adviser to the nation to improve health.

Patient-centered care (PCC): Care that focuses on the patient that is a measure of high-quality health care.

Patient-centered medical home (PCMH): A model of primary care based on holistic patient centeredness and a team approach for the delivery of care.

Pay-for-performance (P4P): A strategy to enhance health care delivery that depends on the utilizing market or purchaser power. Subject to the framework, P4P are financial incentives that financially compensate providers for reaching a range of payer goals (i.e., delivery productivities, data submission measures to a payer, and enhanced quality and patient well-being) (Ramano, Hussey, and Ritley, 2010).

12. *Patient alignment care teams (PACT):* A model of primary care used at the Veterans Administration that has the same concepts of holistic patient-centered care and team-based approach to care as PCMH.

Scope

The investigator used a non-experimental quantitative approach to guide the capstone project. Archival secondary data for patients' satisfaction scores over two consecutive years 2012 and 2013, were extracted from the CAHPS database and compared with PCMH implemented facilities across four regions. The data were analyzed to determine if there was relationship between the two variables. The four retrospective periods of time were compared with four regions (northern, southern, eastern, and western) to determine if there was a trend in the patients' satisfaction data that can be used to make informed decisions for improving patients' satisfaction with their care. The sample consisted of adults 18 years old and older who were seen by their health care provider at least once in within a 12-month period in 2012 and 2013. Target population was 50,000. The investigator took a simple random sample (srs) by running Proc Survey select within the Statistical Analysis Software (SAS). The process for running Proc Survey select is as follows: Proc Survey select data=CAHPS method=srs n = 25000 out=SCAHPS; Run; The Proc Survey select statistic then extracted the simple random sample of 25000 subjects from the CAHPS dataset for each year analyzed (2012 and 2013). The CAHPS dataset then outputted that data sample into a dataset called Sample CAHPS (SCAHPS). The SCAHPS dataset was then randomized and ready for later analysis. The correlation coefficient for patients' satisfaction scores and the number of PCMH implemented facilities over a four-year period was then compared by four different regions to determine if there was a trend in the data from years 2010 to 2013 consecutively.

The instrument used for collecting data is the CG-CAHPS Adult Visit survey. An approved vendor via telephone, electronic mail, or regular mail modes administers the CG-CAPHS survey within six weeks of patients' visits (CAHPS, 2011). Version 2.0 covers 2012 and 2013, for which the PCMH model of care was implemented in regions across the U.S. Surveys are tracked by the assignment of a tracking number at the time the survey is fielded. The investigator did not have direct contact with any of the subjects for this project,

Jacquelene S. Hamer-McGhee, DNP, MSA, RN

nor were the subjects identified. The CAHPS data is publicly available information located on the CMS, AHRQ and NCQA websites.

Limitations

The first limitation for this capstone project was the amount of time between the patient's visit and the patient's completion of the survey. Surveys were administered to patients two to six weeks from the time of the visit. A second limitation was that aggregate data examined from the national CAHPS database were not specific to any one health care group or facility. Therefore, identifying high or low performing organizations based on implementation of PCMH, patient satisfaction scores, health care outcomes, and level of accessibility to health care are beyond the scope of this project. The third limitation exists for the combination of health care facilities in 2012 and 2013 because there is a possibility that they were not the same facilities. Lastly, the project's primary focus was on patient responses from geographical standpoint.

Summary

PCMH is a monumental shift and a precursor to patient satisfaction in today's health care environment. Health care providers are experiencing changes in the way primary care is delivered. Delivering health care is no longer physician driven. The focus is now on the patient and how best to engage the person in their individualized health care *(Alexander & Bae, 2012; Bleich, Osaltin, & Murray, 2009; CMS, 2014; Egger, Day, Scammon, Wilson, & Magill, 2012).*

CHAPTER 2
Literature Review

Introduction

The literature search for this capstone project used the terms Patient-Centered Care (PCC), patient satisfaction, and patient-centered medical home (PCMH) to search the American Sentinel University Library Service, online searches using Google, and Google Scholar. Literature selected included government reports, textbooks, original studies, evaluation of existing literature, past literature reviews, and meta-analysis. Various agencies were used to retrieve information; these agencies include Agency for Healthcare Research and Quality (AHRQ), Centers for Medicare & Medicaid Services (CMS), Department of Health & Human Services (DHHS), and the National Committee for Quality Assurance (NCQA). The Consumer of Health Assessment of Providers and Systems (CHAPS) literature, reports, and handbooks were reviewed. Narrowing the search required a focus on access to care and patient satisfaction that yielded 85 articles. Further research uncovered qualitative, quantitative, mixed, and concept analysis studies. A comprehensive culmination of the literature review is presented below.

Long life expectancy and chronic illness have become urgent concerns for America's health care industry. So much so, the safety and quality of health care have reached a state of critical weakness among the general population (McHugh, Arnold, & Buschman, 2012). This state of critical weakness is largely due to the baby boomer population living longer with chronic illnesses. Additionally, the rapid increase of people 65 years of age and older is expected to grow from 39 million in 2008 to over 69 million in 2030 (AOA, 2014). This change in census will have an enormous impact on health care resources and the ability to deliver safe, quality-focused

Jacquelene S. Hamer-McGhee, DNP, MSA, RN

patient care. Although it is expected that this age group will present with at least three or more comorbidities, the literature and specific health care reported metrics still paint a dim picture for how this rapid growth will affect the delivery and cost of health care (McHugh et al., 2012).

According to The Robert Wood Johnson an Institute of Medicine (IOM) report (2014), *The Future of Nursing*, leading policymakers, health care leaders, health care providers, regulators, purchasers, and others in the health care industry are not well prepared for the influx of chronically ill patients. They are faced with the arduous challenge of how to approach this issue on a global, national, and state level. These health care professionals are also challenged with how to develop and apply viable solutions and strategies that will not only fix the aging population dilemma, but also increase the quality of care and level of patient satisfaction set before them by the Patient Protection and Affordable Care Act.

The problem of a weak health care system does not end with quality and patient satisfaction; health care professionals also struggle with how to keep the escalating cost of health care down while meeting the expectations of their patients for consistent and trusted quality patient-centered care (Greene et al., 2012). Quality of care concerns have escalated since the 1990s with obvious and unexplained variations in the ratio of health care consumption to clinical outcomes across the nation (Alexander & Bae, 2012; Cromwell, Trisolini, Pope, Mitchell, & Greenwald, 2011; Hobbs, 2009; Rosland et al., 2012).

These unexplained variations have also highlighted questions about the traditional approach of health care delivery where the physician delivers health care solo to an individual instead of a team of health care professionals who deliver care to a population of patients. Reinerstsen, Gosfield, Rupp, and Whittington (2007) explained why physicians were having a hard time transitioning from the solo mindset of delivering care by mentioning that the physicians' concentrated efforts are on their profession, their practice, and their personal way of delivering quality care. This traditional structure for delivering health care is considered to be outdated and jepordizes quality of care within a PCMH environment (Reinerstsen et al., 2007).

In the beginning of 2000, reports were published on the issue of the extensive problems associated with safe quality care. The most noteworthy came from the IOM and the RAND Corporation (Cromwell et al., 2011). In 2001, the IOM published *Crossing the Quality Chasm* in 2001, which laid the foundation for redesigning a health care system for 21st-century America and specifically endorsed the President's Advisory Commission statement of purpose (Berwick, 2002).

Background

The face of health care has rapidly changed since the IOM published *Crossing the Quality Chasm* in 2001. From Carlstrom and Ekman's (2012) perspective, health care systems across the globe face challenges to meet the complexity of elevated health care costs and treatment needs for an increasing population of patients with chronic disorders. Past methods and strategies for maintaining a robust health care organization have slowly trickled away. Health care leaders are now expected to take what is left and function with new technology, innovation, and culture changes for today's consumers of care. To meet this challenge, realignment of health care systems' structure and outdated clinical processes must take effect in organizations to accommodate chronic care management as an essential health care goal of the PCMH model (Carlstrom & Ekman, 2012).

To start the process of changing outdated clinical processes and realignment of health care systems, patients were given a new bill of rights through the comprehensive health reform bill and the Patient Protection Affordable Care Act (PPACA), which was signed into law March 23, 2010

(Rozenblum et al., 2013). Since the passing of the comprehensive health reform bill and the PPACA in 2010, there is an increased urgency for improved primary care models, access to care, and patient satisfaction initiatives. Even though the lack of patient engagement, low patient satisfaction scores, and poor access to care continued to elevate health care costs and produce unacceptable health care outcomes, hospital administrators and health care providers continued to overlook the importance of a structured plan to improve customer service and patient satisfaction (Rozenblum et al., 2013).

Becker (2013) and Greene et al. (2012) make good arguments for patient-centered care and patient satisfaction in that health care executives have not directed all aspects of their operational and clinical resources towards placing the patient in the center of health care delivery. Patient-centeredness and customer service are critical elements of a PCMH structure that health care leaders must embrace and understand to ensure this same message reaches those expected to deliver patient-centered care. The support and action of all health care professionals for patient-centered care is essential to maximize patient satisfaction, communication, clinical workflow processes, and resources that support the new structure throughout the organization (Tremblay et al., 2014).

Evidence of little to no patient-centered care or customer service is manifested in patients' frequent use of the emergency room because of the unavailability of same day appointments with assigned health care providers. Readmissions to the hospital in less than 30 days from date of discharge because of poor communication and lack of discharge instructions are results of poor patient-centered care. To address these issues, the Hospital Consumer Assessment of Healthcare Providers & Systems (HCAHPS) surveys were designed to report-patients' satisfaction scores and measures for in-patients. The measures reported for

HCAHPS include: nurse and physician communication with the patient; patient receipt of timely care, pain control, explaination of medication, cleanliness of patient environment, noise control at night, and explaination of care provided.

For this project, the focus is on CAHPS surveys to measure patient satisfaction in the outpatient clinician and group practice environments. The HCAHPS and CAHPS surveys are related in that they both are designed to capture the patients' experience with health care and patient satisfaction. An additional similarity is that these examples of patient-centered care and health care access are believed to be directly linked to barriers of care and poor health care outcomes (IOM, 2012).

Barriers that are believed to cause low patient satisfaction scores and poor access to care include: inadequate staffing for the clinic or in-patient care setting; staff burnout; non-availablity of appointments for scheduling; poor communication between providers and with patients; poor language translation; lack of health care insurance; low economic status; and disparities targeted at ethnicity, age, and gender (IOM, 2012) . According to Patel et al. (2013), the PCMH model proposes an innovative holistic approach to care that maximizes the communication, resources, and clinical processes needed to increase satisfaction scores and access to health care services. However, some researchers believe that the staffing requirements to implement and sustain this stucture have not been well defined and has caused leaders of health care organizations to hesitate with full implementation of PCMH (Patel et al., 2013).

Patient Centered Medical Home

A Patient Centered Medical Home is a practice model predicated on how a practice organizes its operations to better support patients' experiences (Tremblay et al., 2014). Health care professionals have at their disposal theoretical primary care solutions to correct this high cost, low value dilemma, but struggle with how to implement, sustain, and measure a PCMH model of care. Ramano et al. (2010) contended that the amount of capital required to fund health care in the U.S. during 2007 exceeded $2.2 trillion dollars, (16% of the gross domestic product). In addition, the observations of various studies attributed the unexplained variations in quality to underutilization, overutilization, and inappropriate use of health care resources that have led to high mortality and morbidity rates. Part of a health care organization's obligation is to provide appropriate patient-centered care, access that minimizes mortality and morbidity rates, and regulation of the use of medical and human resources.

Literature points to shared themes of appropriate access to care, team-based approach to care, augmented electronic medical record use, planned care, and empowered patient self-management. All these principles provide the foundation for the primary care models of PCMH, Patient Alignment Teams (PACT), and Care by Design (CBD). According to Egger et al., (2012), CBD is focused on the process of primary care practice formation while the standards for PCMH focus on structure.

Supporters of PCMH contend that access to care improvement processes rely on the adaptation of this primary care model for delivering quality and efficient care (Schwenk, 2014). Schwenk (2014) has a different view for the efficiency of PCMH and mentioned a project conducted by Friberg that did not yield much of a return on investment after three years of participating in a pilot study. The study revealed one chronic disease quality improvement measure out of 11 where a nephrology service monitored patients for diabetes.

With the passing of the ACA, health care leaders discussed providing coverage for the uninsured. Pointed attempts to provide care for this population brought to light innovative practice models. Health care leaders agreed that simply providing coverage for all would not solve the cost, access, and quality issues that plague the U.S. system of health care. Health care leaders shifted their focus to providing lower costs care and to improving patient care while enhancing both providers and patients' satisfaction. The PCMH model has emerged as a comprehensive delivery model that works on both regional and state levels to control costs, coordinate care, and improve satisfaction and outcomes (Patient Care Collaborative, 2009).

The Patient Centered Medical Home is a not a new concept. It was originally developed by a group of pediatric physicians, the American Academy of Pediatrics (AAP), in the 1960s as a concept of primary care to better manage chronically ill pediatric patients. It was not until the 1980s that PCMH was introduced to manage chronically ill adults. Today, along with AAP, the transformed vision of a patient-centered medical home is also advocated by the American Academy of Family Physicians, American College of Physicians, and American Osteopathic Association (Wexler, 2012).

A Patient Centered Medical Home is defined as an integration model of care utilized in the primary care setting that strives to deliver quality, cost-effective non-fragmented care (Marshall et al., 2011). According to Marshall et al. (2011), the PCMH model promotes stronger patient-provider relationships using a team-based approach to increase continuity of patient care between providers and increased access to health services. However, there was no mention of patient satisfaction in relation to stronger patient-provider relationships. Results form the Nelson project highlighted the significance in patients' satisfaction, which was higher in Veterans Administration (VA) facilities with successful implementation of PACT versus those without the successful implementation experience (Nelson et al., 2014).

The Veterans Health Administration (VHA) started the process of transforming its settings for health care delivery through planned change where the VHA culture experienced major transformation upon building its PACT in the 1990s. Process of care was evident through the implementation of comprehensive electronic medical records, performance measurement, and improvement programs such as clinical outcome goals for glycemic and hypertension control for patients with diabetic and cancer screenings (Rosland et al., 2012).

Today, the VHA is a regionally integrated system focused on outpatient primary care. The Patient Alignment Care Team initiative was constructed by incorporating the PCMH model of care for the VHA. In their project on VHA facilities, Rosland et al.'s (2012) used elements of the Donabedian framework (structure, access, and health care outcomes). Nelson et al., 2014 illustrated the effectiveness of PACT before and after implementation by measuring patients' satisfaction, quality of care, staff burnout, and hospital emergency department use. Nelson et al. focused on developing a comprehensive tool called the PACT Implementation Progress Index, Pi2 that would not cause undue problems for the respondents of their survey.

Patient Centered Care

In 2001, the Institute of Medicine report *Crossing the Quality Chasm* heightened the public's awareness of patient-centered care. Patient centeredness became a high priority on the nation's agenda and triggered health care administrators to pay close attention to surveys and public reports that measure patient satisfaction and patient experiences. Rozenblum et al. (2013) illustrated how patient-centered care improved patients' expectations and improved clinical outcomes. Health care organizations around the world strive to become more patient oriented and use patient surveys to assess their progress for improving patient-centered care (Rozenblum et al., 2013).

Several studies found that health care organizations that succeed in fostering patient-centered care in their organizations incorporated it as a strategic objective. Researchers also found that leaders at all levels need to be committed to and engaged in active measurement and feedback of patiet satisfaction as well as engagement of patients and staff (Rozenblum et al., 2013). Studies report that the main determinants of patient satisfaction are associated with clinician behavior, including communication with patients' concerns and needs and involvement of patients in decision making.

Patient-centered care has drawn increasing interest in recent years, highlighting the importance of incorporating patients' needs and perspectives into care delivery. Consistent with this notion, implementation of patient-centered care and higher patient satisfaction has been shown to be associated with improved clinical outcomes and health service efficiency and has a positive effect on business metrics (Rozenblum et al., 2013). Berwick (2002) contended that patient satisfaction and patient-centered care should be the fundamental sources for the definition of quality in health care.

The Institute of Medicine defines patient-centered care, as cited by Greene (2012), as "care that is respectful of and responsive to individual patient preferences, needs and values" (p. 49). This means there are several characteristics to consider in relation to patients' health care experiences and goal-oriented outcomes. Bensing's description of Patient-Centered Care (PCC), (as cited by Greene, 2012), is one of a "container concept" that encompasses many different characteristics of behavior. The dimensions and characteristics of Green's (2012) PCC conceptual framework to cooperatively influence patients' health care experiences include: (a) interpersonal dimension (relationship), communication, knowing the patients, and the importance of teams; (b) clinical dimension (provision of care), including clinical decision support, coordination and continuity, and types of encounters; and (c) structural dimensions (system features), composed of a built environment, access to care, and information technology.

Hobbs (2009) viewed PCC throughout the clinical research as inconsistent and difficult to implement. Green (2012) echoed the difficulty for implementing PCC but attributed the complexity to the daily multidimensional workflow process. Health care providers struggle with when and how to manage the clinical dynamics of PCC delivery for every fluctuating patient encounter throughout the day. The constant fluctuations cause barriers for the consistency of integrating PCC into daily workflow processes. Examples of fluctuation throughout the day may be attributed to staffing shortages, electronic health record downtime, environmental factors, or the patient's needs being too difficult to meet in the short amount of time allotted for the patient encounter.

From a nursing perspective, Lusk and Fater (2013) argued that PCC is not clearly defined in the health care community based their manuscript on a synthesis of literature to reveal which constructs define PCC and how delivery of PCC affects patient health care outcomes. Lusk and Fater (2013) defined PCC as:

The provision of care incorporating contextural elements and including the attributes of encoraging patient autonomy, attitude of the nurse, and individualizing patient care by the nurse. Behaviors that bridge the gaps for the provison of PCC include communicating, listening, treating the patient as a unique individual, respect values, and promptly respond to the patient needs.

The IOM contended that PCC is a foundation that needed for high-quality, safe care to be available and delivered to all patients. PCC should also focus on meeting the patients' needs and expectations for non-fragmented care. Wexler, King, and Andrews (2012) found that the only way to deliver patient-centered care is to individualize patient desires and needs and place them at the center of care. Improved care coordination and increased access are parts of a larger whole. As the PCMH process evolves, it is important to incorporate patients' opinions for educating residents and students about PCMH care, as well as design how care is delivered. Results from Wexler et al.'s project were consistent with other studies reporting consistent coordinated care and access to health care services, all of which patients believe are the foundational elements critical to the PCMH model of care (IOM, 2012; Nelson et al., 2010; Rosland et al., 2013).

In their qualitative project, Wexler et al. (2012) discussed how patients exhibited strong opinions about care coordination, patient self-management, and availability of appointments as the top priorities for PCMH. More work in the U.S. is required to adequately process and implement standards designed to measure and improve patients' satisfaction and quality of care. To date, various in-depth studies have examined whether patient-centered care influences improving health care outcomes such as diabetes, asthma, hypertension, and patient satisfaction.

The literature exposed studies focused on developing actionable conceptual frameworks for patient-centered care (Green et al., 2012; Hobbs, 2009; Lusk & Fater, 2013). Studies reviewed included patient engagement, staff engagement, and primary care models such as patient-centered medical home and patient alignment care teams (Alexander & Bae, 2012; Baker et al.; Egger et al., 2012; Nelson et al., 2014; Rosland, et al., 2012; Wexler, 2012;). Methods used for the studies throughout the literature review included quantitative, quantitative, descriptive analysis, conceptualization, case project methodology, exploratory, explanatory, and descriptive. Other pilot studies uncovered statistical significance for the implementation of PCMH using frameworks, such as Donabedian and IOM.

Accountable Care Organization (ACO)

Jacquelene S. Hamer-McGhee, DNP, MSA, RN

Policymakers on the national stage recognized the need for accountable care, a term that has a vision for greater value than the current system delivers. Discussion is currently progressing to fit the PCMH model into the support structure that is achieved through Accountable Care Organizations (ACO). An ACO is a provider-led entity that is willing to manage the full continuum of care and be accountable for the overall costs and quality of care for a defined population (Spooner et al., 2012). Like the PCMH, ACOs incorporate accountable care into the trusted relationship patients have with their primary care providers. The PCMH and the ACO work to complement each other for the delivery of and transformation of health care while decreasing costs and enhancing quality (Spooner et al., 2012). Built on the foundation of the PCMH, ACOs provide the essential delivery system infrastructure beyond primary care practice to realize the PCMH model (Patient Care Collaborative, 2009).

Investment Required to Implement PCMH

In comparison, Paustian et al. (2013) demonstrated relationships between a PCMH model implementation, higher quality of care, and reduced cost of care. Based on the initial assessment, the project supports continued investment in PCMH implementation but states that if cost savings and quality improvement relationships observed in this study were to be reinforced by additional evaluations of the PCMH model, additional financial support for PCMH implementation may be needed. As demonstrated in Donabedian's framework under structure of care, structure presents a significant challenge for many primary care practices and clinics with substantial investments of time and expenses. If these added resources require primary care practices and clinics to take on the investments alone, their attitudes towards PCMH implementation may be relentlessly minimized (Paustian et al., 2013).

A study conducted by Patel et al. (2013) concluded that full PCMH implementation required an elevation of a practice's staffing and function roles as well as an evaluation of the needs for its population. This study was also in keeping with Paustian et al.'s (2013) position on the significant investments of time and capital associated with the augmentation of technology and staffing ratios. Patel et al. (2013) noted that achievement of the goal to improve outcomes and better care comes at a price of additional staffing with a required increase of expertise and training. While prospective long-term savings from implementation of PCMH could possibly compensate for the additional upfront cost of increased staffing, more research is required along with additional funding sources to recognize full PCMH return on investment (ROI) (Patel et al., 2013).

According to Patel et al. (2013), the PCMH staffing structure was not clear, so they sought to evaluate the roles of personnel within the PCMH model and then proposed an appropriate staffing ratio based on the results and associated incremental costs to implement this model of care. Findings revealed that 4.25 support personnel were needed for everyone physician full-time equivalent (FTE) (Patel et al., 2013). The base case model for PCMH is 2.68 support personnel per one physician FTE that revealed a 59% increase (Patel et al., 2013). A sensitivity analysis was conducted to test validity of interview data collected. The results revealed 1.57 per FTE (Patel et al., 2013). Patel et al. (2013) contended that their study suggested the need for additional staff with specific expertise and training to implement a PCMH model. Further studies on the opportunities for funding additional staffing costs are needed to realize the full potential of the PCMH model of care.

Staffing within primary care is challenging. The primary care staffing model could positively benefit from incorporating more nurse practitioners (NPs) into the PCMH model care (Naylor & Kurtzman, 2010). Naylor and Kurtzman (2010) reported that 70-80% of advanced practice nurses' work in primary care and are available to fill the gaps of lost physician providers. The augmentation of NPs into the PCMH arena holds a high potential for savings on resource allocations while adding value. Most of the literature reviewed on costing in the PCMH model of care focused on physician staffing with clinical support personnel (such as registered nurses and licensed practical nurses). The hidden potential for improving all aspects of primary care, especially access and patient satisfaction, are intentionally glossed over (Naylor & Kurtzman, 2010; IOM, 2012).

In their study, Naylor and Kurtzman (2010) recommended study that policy makers, the public, and other health care stakeholders take a deeper look at the growth of the chronically ill and elderly populations. Stakeholders need to act quickly and understand the urgency to fill the gaps in health care quality and increased spending. The demand for high-quality primary care services will continue along with a decline in physician primary care population. Given this decline in primary care physicians, it appears to be a promising future for nursing in primary care. Naylor and Kurtzman (2010) contended, "The contributions of nurse practitioners are a vital step toward achieving high-value health care"

Patient Satisfaction

Accomplishing high levels of patient satisfaction involves hospital management acceptance and participation in patient-centered care progress initiatives. Hospital leadership is also expected to engage frontline clinicians in this process (Rozenblum et al., 2013). However, additional investigation is necessary to determine to what degree new primary care models, such as PCMH, affect patient satisfaction, patient health care outcomes, improved access to care between variations of practice types, and increased patient engagement (Paustian et al., 2013).

The Center for Advancing Health Behavior defines patient engagement as patient initiative toward receiving the most value from accessible health care services (Oldenburg, 2013). The center explained the difference between patient engagement and compliance by noting that compliance means conformity to a health care provider's directive, while engagement encompasses patients' involvement in the processes of their health care and the acceptance of professional health care advice (Oldenburg, 2013).

The PCMH approach to managing chronic illness is believed to increase patients' satisfaction and improve access to care for patients who are categorized in both the acute and chronic care categories. Health care providers can accomplish more by taking on the role of overseeing and coaching their staff members care for chronically ill patients using innovative tools such as communication through secure messaging, telemedicine, and providing 24-hour service through a nurse advice line. Other PCMH tools for increasing patient satisfaction and enhancing access to care include mobile health devices and tele-pharmacy.

Timely Appointments/Access to care

Communication problems and access to care barriers involving a shortage of health care provider support present unique struggles for organizations. When there is a shortage of providers in the primary care environment, patients are unable to establish a rapport with their providers, which interferes with the health care providers' ability to render care that is coordinated and individualized for their patients. Physician shortages cause physician health care providers to leave the primary care discipline to pursue other options (IOM, 2012).

Physicians are being held to a much higher standard than nurse practitioners and physician assistants through the Affordable Care Act (ACA), and tighter regulations mandated by CMS for reimbursement, such as pay for performance (P4P) operational models. This is a model of reimbursement for health care providers based on how well they perform their responsibilities of ensuring quality health care for their patients. Many physicians have found this model of reimbursement difficult to manage, and as a result, have had to leave their private practices and seek employment with hospitals and other health care facilities (IOM, 2012). Even worse, some have had to exit primary care altogether and seek different disciplines or retire depending on how long they were in the profession.

Another reason for staffing problems associated with access to care and timely appointments is attributed to low graduation rates for primary care residents. Residents are choosing to move away from the primary care discipline and specialize in other options (IOM, 2012). From a business angle, the lack of primary care fellows has affected the primary care panel sizes, so much so that the phenomenon has attracted the attention of the American Medical Association and motivated the organization to start incentivizing residents through the promotion of primary care opportunities. The primary care promotion is an effort to increase panel sizes and patient enrollment into health care plans.

Patel et al. (2013) noted that staffing ratios for full-time equivalent (FTE) providers functioning in PCMH environments on average have panel sizes ranging from 625-2500. Panel sizes are of concern for physicians in the process of or currently operating in a PCMH model. Patel et al. (2013) and Schwenk (2014) contended that because of the daily balancing act needed for staffing a PCMH environment, difficulties arise when there are not enough providers to handle the workload. This workload problem can quickly transform into an access to care, patient satisfaction, or clinical outcome problem. Chronically ill patients' emergency department visits are a result of them being recently hospitalized without the ability to obtain follow-up appointments with their primary care providers that same day (IOM, 2012).

According to information revealed in AHRQ, the non-availability of appointments is one of the top issues that results in patients' dissatisfaction (AHRQ, 2014). Patients are particularly disappointed with the need to repeat their health problems to several different providers. Nielsen (2014) emphasized that a chronically ill patient, on average, will experience up to 20 different providers, to include a mixture of primary and specialty care consultations. Fragmented care for chronically ill patients is the catalyst for skyrocketing health care costs in the U.S. and the main cause for poor health care outcomes and decreased patient satisfaction (Nielsen, 2014).

Physicians can expect an increase in previously uninsured patients with chronic illnesses after the passing of the Affordable Care Act (Schwenk, 2014), which mandates that every American enroll in a health care plan. The increase of previously uninsured patients translates into an increase of chronic care management, as these patients do not regularly present to the hospital for preventative care. Individuals often

Jacquelene S. Hamer-McGhee, DNP, MSA, RN

wait until signs and symptoms of illness are so far advanced that the disease is very difficult to manage (IOM, 2012). Health care providers see this influx of patients as an overwhelming problem and are under a great deal of pressure as they face this problem in addition to new mandates and regulations (CMS, 2014; Nelson et al., 2014). Health care providers often feel they will burn out from trying to monitor chronic care, increase patient satisfaction, and improve patient health care outcomes (Schwenk, 2014; Carlstrom & Ekman, 2012).

The shortage of primary care staff and burnout problems are not subject to physicians alone.

There is also a shortage of nurse practitioners (NPs) and physician assistants (PAs) in the primary care environment. This is although nurse practitioner and physician assistant training programs are shorter and produce far more health care providers than physicians' programs (IOM, 2012). Nurse practitioners and physician assistants can easily fill the shortage gaps and increase the availability of appointments to help decrease the effects of limited access to care and dissatisfied patients (IOM, 2012). Even though the NP and PA health care provider assets are more available, health care administrators overlook the value of staffing their primary care environments with NPs and PAs. The expectation for health care providers overall is to consistently deliver and maintain optimal patient satisfaction scores, while improving the quality of patient-centered care that will continue to grow (Patel et al., 2013).

Physicians will no longer be able to work solo under the new health care reform requirements. They will need a well-structured plan for implementation of a new primary care model (such as PCMH) and the help of a support team to meet the demands of delivering patient centered care to chronically ill patients, engaging patients in their care, and ensuring accurate documentation, all within a 20-minute encounter (Rozenblum et al., 2013). An example of a PCMH support team would consist of registered nurses, licensed practical nurses, nurse assistants, or super techs (certified nurse assistants with the responsibility of conducting administrative tasks), a registered dietician, pharmacist, social worker, case manager, and a clinic practice manager (Patel et al., 2013, Pausitan et al., 2013). The logistical resources and training requirements for the development of a plan are other aspects of PCMH implementation that health care administrators do not initially consider, add to that a shortage of support staff and space to accommodate the employees (See Appendix A).

Health Care Provider Ratings

Health care system responsiveness specifically refers to the manner and environment in which people are treated when they seek health care (Bleich et al., 2009). It is important that health care providers maintain ratings that meet or exceed the industry standards. Meeting these standards is important because providers are often judged by their leaders according to their ratings. A study conducted by Bottone, Musich, and Wang (2014) on the report of high satisfaction and positive experiences with care for older obese adults found that compared to patients in the normal weight category, obese patients ratings reported higher satisfaction than patients in the normal weight category. Obese patients in this project also received personal recommendations from their providers on preventive measures as opposed to non-obese patients.

Patient-centered care was apparent when obese patients experienced an office visit with their providers and participated in a conversation at least three or more times in less than 6 months. The level of care and attention required to care for patients with this comorbidity automatically creates an atmosphere for increased dyad communication between the provider and patient. This level of communication contributes to high levels of provider ratings (Bleich, 2009).

Jacquelene S. Hamer-McGhee, DNP, MSA, RN

It has become apparent that patient satisfaction reports are what drive the health care industry. Since the passing of legislation such The Excellent Care for All Bill in Ontario Canada and the Affordable Care Act in the U.S, it was mandated by public health care administrations that hospitals conduct yearly patient satisfaction surveys. Outcomes from these surveys set the foundation for performance enhancement programs, which in turn determine the quality improvement metrics health care executives are responsible for meeting. These quality metrics established by the government, incentivize those providers who can maintain a level of sustainment for meeting the metrics established for reimbursement (Detsky & Shaul, 2013).

Like the government law in Canada, the U.S. operates under The Affordable Care Act. However, the reimbursement incentive process is slightly different in the 1% of reimbursements authorized by Medicare to be taken away from health care facilities with low patient satisfaction scores and given to health care facilities with higher achievement levels. Detsky and Shaul (2013) argued that patient-centered care is not what it seems and that incentives should be apparent for both the provider sas well as the patients. Patients have taken the patient-centered care to another level and have started to demand or expect providers to deliver patient-directed care (Detsky & Shaul, 2013).

Patient-directed care is simply an expectation from the patients that the physicians would give them whatever they want. For instance, patients may feel that because they have completed a round of antibiotics while in an outpatient status, they would need a follow-up lab tests to ensure the medication was effective. However, complying with such demands may cause the provider to deviate away from the clinical practice guidelines to avoid negative feedback on patient satisfaction surveys.

According to a study conducted by Greene, Hibbard, Sacks, and Overton (2013), a different perspective of patient-centered care is described.   The study focused on the relationship between health care providers and patient activation.   Patient activation is a concept that incorporates how much knowledge patients have about their health care and their skill sets, which gives them the confidence to communicate with their provider on a deeper level of engagement (Hibbard & Green, 2013).

The more activated patients are in their care, the better the outcomes are for satisfaction (Green, 2013).   This combination of transnationalism allows the providers or practices to meet or exceed metrics set by governmental agencies.

Communication

Just as providers can accomplish more by taking on a more focused leadership role within the PCMH model, they could also see the same level of accomplishment with their patients through active communication. The following patient satisfaction needs were brought to the forefront in Wexler et al.'s (2012) perspective on communication and coordination of care:

1. Health care providers must change their expectations for patient compliance and attentively listen and anticipate non-verbal clues that encourage patients to participate with in a negotiated plan for their care.

2. All providers of care commit to following a framework built to engage patients as individuals.

3. Health care administrators provide integrated clinical systems that allow patients to access their health information and obtain the knowledge required to embrace engagement of a healthier life through care-plans and processes designed to educate.

4. Health care providers empower and equip patients with the tools and education that enhance their access to care and communication with their health care team. It is imperative for

these tools and services to feel comfortable enough for the patients to comprehend and incorporate into their behavioral changes.

Helpful and Courteous Staff

A State Board of Nursing study found that almost 50% of the complaints reported by patients originated from rude, offensive, and less than helpful behavior by health care staff (Brennan & Monson, 2014). The litigation for these complaints proves to be more costly than malpractice suits and pose an elevated risk for safety problems such as medication and medical errors. Brennan and Monson (2014) stated "Professionalism is an indispensable element in the compact between the medical profession and society that is based on trust and places the needs of patients above all other circumstances"

In their study, Brennan and Monson (2014) focused on revealing attributes and responsibilities that foster an organizational team-based culture of professionalism. Patients expect that everyone on their health care team would function as a unit to deliver the best possible care. They tend to trust that each member of the team is expertly trained to perform their specific job (McLaughlin & Kaluzny, 2006). Brennan and Monson (2014) mentioned how important it is to strategize positive values and inter-professional relationships through alignment of organizational systems and structures.

Patients remain loyal to an organization when they trust their physicians and health care teams (Brennan & Monson, 2014; Furlow, 2014). In fact, studies reveal that patients who have this level of trust often seek the care needed and reveal personal information about their health history. This rapport between patients and health care providers sets a foundation for committed patients who follow through with recommended treatment plans and subsequent follow-up appointments. From a business standpoint, the level of patients' commitment is important because regulators tie the outcomes of patient care to reimbursement of the health care provided.

When physicians and health care staff approach patients with harsh undertones and an air of superiority, they open themselves up to costly lawsuits and adverse or sentinel events. Studies have shown that patients are more forgiving and less likely to file a lawsuit when physicians and health care staff "go the extra mile" to ensure the patients' needs and unique desires are met or exceeded. Helpful and courteous attention towards patients is non-existent in the presence of staff burnout (Brennan & Monson, 2014). A few incidences that are likely to cause staff burnout stem from frustration with policies and procedures that force elevated working expectations, fostering a culture of degradation of character and bullying. These destructive characteristics cause barriers and lessen the providers' and health care professionals' ability to advocate on behalf of patients (Brennan & Monson, 2014). Organizational staff must be held responsible for their obligation to be respectful and helpful to both patients and each other.

Conclusion

The Joint Principles for the Medical Education of Physicians as cited by Patel et al. (2013) noted that the goal of primary care is to replace intermittent care with synchronized anticipatory, team-based care. However, team-based care and fully implementing Patient Centered Medical Homes requires more than just following a set of guidelines.

Achieving the ultimate goals of increasing patient satisfaction and access to care essentially means upfront costs for increased numbers of qualified staffing with the required proficiency and training. It would take additional studies, funding sources, and a few years to see the tangible and intangible long-term savings related to the implementation of PCMH and increased costs for staffing (Patel et al., 2013). To that end, the organization will first need to embrace the changed concept of patient-centered care (Carlstrom & Ekman, 2012).

Jacquelene S. Hamer-McGhee, DNP, MSA, RN

In a patient-centered environment, patients are encouraged and empowered to participate in their health care and to build confidence and make better choices for a healthier lifestyle. Patient-centered care assures each patient is treated with dignity, privacy, and confidentiality.

Summary

Leaders in the health care community exhibit strong opinions about care coordination, patient self-management, and improved access to care as the top priorities for PCMH (Wexler et al., 2012). More work is needed in the U.S. to adequately process and implement standards designed to measure and improve patients' satisfaction and quality of care through the implementation of patient-centered care and the PCMH model of care. Various in-depth studies have examined the question of whether patient-centered care influences improving health care outcomes for patients with diabetes, asthma, and hypertension and increasing patients' satisfaction. The literature review revealed studies focused on developing actionable conceptual frameworks for patient-centered care (Green, 2012; Hobbs, 2009; Lusk & Fater, 2013).

Methods used for the studies throughout the literature review included quantitative, quantitative, descriptive analysis, conceptualization, case project methodology, exploratory, explanatory, and descriptive. Other pilot studies uncovered statistical significance for the implementation of PCMH using frameworks, such as Donabedian and IOM.

Patients' satisfaction significantly decreases when there are no available appointments, long wait times in the physician's offices, the pharmacy, and other ancillary services. In fact, when there is a shortage of staff, patients may experience degradation in customer service, which also decreases the level of patients' satisfaction scores. Other factors that decrease patients' satisfaction are fragmented communication of care between providers, poor communication with the patients, and staffing shortages that cause provider ratings to slide below the normal industry standard. More effort is required to ensure that patients' satisfaction scores are at least within the acceptable industry level.

Chapter 3 provides a brief summary of the Capstone project's methodology. Details about the quantitative secondary analysis design will explain the statistical analysis of patients' satisfaction responses throughout the U.S. across four different regions.

CHAPTER 3
Methods

Introduction

This project examined the relationship between patients' satisfaction scores and the number of Patient Centered Medical Homes (PCMH) in regions across the U.S. The variables identified were PCMH model and Patients' Satisfaction Scores (PTSAT). Data were extracted from the CAHPS database provided by the CAHPS database administrators. The CAHPS database was accessible through a secure email link for a brief period. Once admitted into the secure link, Statistical Analysis Software (SAS) was downloaded onto a secure computer, followed by a download of the CAHPS data file stored in SAS. The processes for developing, testing for reliability and validity, and fielding the survey instrument are explained in the project design. A brief overview of the sampling guidelines as well as data collection modes is provided later in this chapter.

Project Design

The design for this project was a non-experimental quantitative analysis design utilizing secondary data to determine if there is a relationship between patients' satisfaction scores and the number of PCMH facilities that have been implemented across regions in the U.S. for years 2012 and 2013 consecutively. The investigator extracted de-identified archived survey data from the online public CAHPS database. This project was conducted retrospectively by utilizing patient satisfaction survey results for health care facilities across the U.S. in four different regions (northern, southern, eastern, and western) over four consecutive years (2012 and 2013). Each region was examined to help determine if there are any trends associated with the two variables. The results of the analysis were used to determine if a significant statistical correlation exists between patients' satisfaction scores and the number of PCMH facilities that have been implemented.

Instruments

The CAHPS Survey initiative is a public partnership that originated in 1995 with government support of the Agency for Healthcare Research and Quality (AHRQ). Private research organizations that were involved in the earliest stages of the development of the CAHPS survey products included: The Harvard Medical School in Boston, Massachusetts, the RAND Corporation, a global policy think tank headquartered in Santa Monica, California, and the Research Triangle Institute (RTI), one of the world leading research institutes located in Research Triangle Park, North Carolina (CAHPS, 2011).

According to Hargraves, Hays, and Cleary (2003), revisions for the instrument's validity and reliability have been updated and revised over time. In addition, a plan-level reliability that attains .70 for five composites occurs when there are fewer than 170 replies for each plan. Cronbach's alpha greater than or equal to .75 represents high internal consistency for two of the composites, while Cronbach's alpha ranging from .58 - .62 represents replies for items in three other composites that display less of an internal consistency (Hargraves et al., 2003).

The instrument used for extracting patient satisfaction data was the Consumer Assessment of Healthcare Providers and Systems (CAHPS)-Adult Visit Questionnaire (See Appendix B). The Consumer Assessment of Healthcare Providers and Systems (CAHPS)-Adult Visit Questionnaire is a 31-item survey that captures patients' reports of their health care experiences. The survey includes four composites: (a) getting timely appointments, care, and information; (b) how well providers communicate with patients; (c) helpful, courteous, and respectful office staff; and (d) patient ratings of their providers. Results for the CAHPS surveys are free and publicly available on the NCQA, PCPCC, CMS, and AHRQ websites.

Data Collection, Management, and Analysis Plan

Data analysis for this non-experimental quantitative study used Statistical Analysis Software (SAS) downloaded from a secure email link provided by the CAHPS database administrator upon request to use the dataset for research. Once the request to use the data was accepted a signed acceptance of use agreement was forwarded to the CAHPS database administrator. The SAS software was used to organize, calculate, and analyze the research data. A simple randomized sample of 50,000 subjects for each region over a two-year period (2012 and 2013) was extracted from the CAHPS database. The patient satisfaction data was examined for outliers, skewness, and kurtosis. Descriptive statistics were used to measure central tendency, measures of variability, and measures of relative standing throughout the project data.

The hypothesis was assessed with a Pearson-r Correlation Coefficient instead of t-test. According to Ha and Ha (2012), correlation coefficient requires that the data used for a project be either interval or ratio scale. Interval variables were used to measure and analyze the correlation coefficient of patients' satisfaction scores and number of PCMH implemented facilities for different regions across the U.S. Correlation coefficient measures the degree to which corresponding scores inhabit the same virtual positions in their distributions (closely related). For instance, it is possible that lower X values correlate with lower Y values called a direct relationship or; the opposite association, where the X values associate with higher Y values (Ha & Ha, 2012).

Jacquelene S. Hamer-McGhee, DNP, MSA, RN

Ha and Ha (2012) provided characteristics for correlation coefficients by noting that correlation values always have a range of strong-negative to strong- positive (-1 and +1). When the coefficient has a positive slope, this indicates and inverse relationship. If the correlation equals zero, this indicates there is no relationship at all among the variables, which supports the null hypothesis. A -1.00 coefficient implies a perfect inverse relationship among variables and a +1.00 implies a perfect direct (positive) relationship among variables.

There is a table for critical values of *r* based on degrees of freedom, which is N-2. N-2 is used verses N-1 because there are two constant variables used to assess the level of variance for both measures concurrently. The investigator chose to use an alpha of 0.05 to find the critical value of *r* at the point where the null hypothesis was rejected. Rejection of the null hypothesis means r was not significantly different from zero. In the instance where the correlation coefficient was not appropriate, the non-parametric test for Spearman's rank order correlation coefficient was appropriate (Ha & Ha, 2012).

All data that were used for this project were archival data and are public information available on the Internet. Subjects were not identifiable, and there was no direct contact with the investigator or with any subjects. Additionally, this project did not involve primary data collection from human subjects. Examination of information is freely available to the public no confidentiality protection is required. The names of the clinician or group practices were not included when describing the data. The data were not collected for analysis until approval from the American Sentinel University (ASU) Institutional Review Board (IRB) was obtained.

Methodology Appropriateness

The non-experimental quantitative research design was appropriate for this project to reveal whether there a

Jacquelene S. Hamer-McGhee, DNP, MSA, RN

correlation between the study variables exists. Additionally, there was no need for identification or establishment of a causality relationship for this design. The investigator did not control the independent variable because it cannot be manipulated after the occurrence (Sharma, 2012).

Another design considered for this capstone project included the ex post facto design, a quantitative design that is used to investigate whether there is a relationship between the variables identified in the project (Sharma, 2012). Even though the ex post facto design does not identify a causative relationship or allow for the control of the independent variable, it is better suited for investigating the correlation of variables instead of investigating a significant statistical difference between the variables. After considering the ex post facto design for quantitative research, quantitative analysis framework was more appropriate. This quantitative design used a systematic process to collect information with an instrument and statistically analyzed it.

This project simply required the examination of a phenomenon by numerically representing observations and statistical analysis (Langford, 2001).

Feasibility and Appropriateness

This project involved minimal cost, support, and services because data were extracted from the Consumer of Health Assessment of Providers and Systems (CAHPS) database at no cost to the investigator as access to the CAHPS survey instrument and database are open to the public on the Medicare website. The data collected from the survey responses were stored in a data repository made available to researchers and sponsors for the purpose of research and benchmarking. Therefore, extracting data from the CAHPS national database was less costly and less time-sensitive than conducting primary research, where each participant would have to be surveyed.

Jacquelene S. Hamer-McGhee, DNP, MSA, RN

Summary

The objective of the project was to determine if there was a correlation between patients' satisfaction scores and PCMH implemented facilities. Chapter 3 provided a summary of the project methodology and how the quantitative design guided the statistical analysis of patients' satisfaction scores for clinician and group practices across four regions of the U.S. for 2012 and 2013. The population for this project was 50,000 patients over the age of 18 and seen in a clinician or group practice at least once throughout the year. A simple randomized sample of 25,000 patient responses in 2012 and 2013 across four regions (North, South, East, and West) was taken from the CAHPS database for analysis. Upon completion of this project, a determination was made that there was a correlation between patients' satisfaction scores and the number of PCMH facilities across the U.S. in four different regions in 2012 and 2013.

Jacquelene S. Hamer-McGhee, DNP, MSA, RN

CHAPTER 4
Findings

Introduction

This project, a retrospective review of patient satisfaction scores and the relationship to Patient Centered Medical Home implementation, examined if increasing the number of facilities with the PCMH model of care influenced patients' experiences reported in the form of patients' satisfaction scores. The investigator examined if there was a relationship between patients' satisfaction scores and the number of PCMH-implemented facilities in four regions of the U.S. for 2012 and 2013.

Patient satisfaction CAHPS data, fielded by an authorized vendor, already existed in the CAHPS database; therefore, subjects were not selected or enlisted to participate in the project. The investigator did not conduct primary research or have contact with any of the subjects. For that reason, the investigator did not need to obtain an informed consent from participants. Patient satisfaction data is publicly available from the CAHPS database free of cost (CAHPS, 2013). Data for this project were extracted from the online database provided by the CAHPS database administration team. There was no risk to participants or health care facilities, and no identifiable patient or health care facility information was obtained.

Purpose of the Project

The purpose of the project was to determine if there was a relationship between the overall CAHPS scores and the number of PCMH facilities by regions in the United States for years 2012 and 2013.

Data Analysis

The investigator used retrospective data from the Consumer of Health Assessment of Providers and Systems (CAHPS) database and extracted patients' satisfaction data during the following periods: January 1, 2012 to December 31, 2012 and January 1, 2013 to December 31, 2013. CAHPS is a public program initiative supported by AHRQ to develop standardized surveys of patients' experiences. The CAHPS instrument is a 12-month questionnaire divided into four composites (access to care, communication, helpful staff, and provider scoring) containing a total of 31 questions to capture and measure patients' satisfaction scores.

The project was conducted under a non-experimental quantitative analysis design that examined the relationship between CAHPS patient satisfaction scores and the number of Patient Centered Medical Home (PCMH) implemented health care facilities across regions of the U.S in 2012 and 2013. No causality relationship was determined for this project. The target populations changed upon receipt of the data files from the CAHPS administrator, as the files were very large. Patient responses captured in the data sets across four regions for the year 2012 were 613,396 and 428,154 for the year 2013. The investigator used 50,000 randomized patients' responses (25,000 from each year) which were a representative sample from the available data files. Inclusions for the sample were patients 18 years and older with at least one outpatient visit with their primary care provider during a 12-month period, If the patient was seen more than once in the 12-month period, the most recent visit was used, and that data was sent to the investigator for inclusion in the study. Exclusion for the sample included de-duplication, which meant only one person per household was included in the sample even though others in the household may have completed a survey. The investigator received the data from the CAHPS administrator de-duplicated, which was

Jacquelene S. Hamer-McGhee, DNP, MSA, RN

in compliance with the data use agreement required by CAHPS. The agreement to keep the data de-duplicated was with health care facilities that provided their patient satisfaction data to the CAHPS database online.

Responses were drawn from the randomized data file which consisted of 25,000 patients' satisfaction responses for each year (2012 and 2013), a total of 50,000 responses from four regions across the U.S. According to the CAHPS definition for region, the regions were listed as: NORTHEAST, MIDWEST, SOUTH, and WEST. The process for creating the randomized database consisted of extracting a Simple Randomized Sample (srs) from the CAHPS database by using syntax language within the Statistical Analysis Software (SAS), version 9.3. The process for running Proc Survey select began with selecting: Proc Survey select data = CAHPS method = srs n = 25000 out = SCAHPS; Run; The Proc Survey select statistic then extracted the srs of 25,000 randomized subjects from the CAHPS dataset. The CAHPS dataset then extracted srs data into a dataset called "Sample CAHPS" (SCAHPS). At this point, the SCAHPS dataset was randomized and ready for data analysis. The variables identified for this project were the number of PCMH facilities (PCMH_CNT), total patients' satisfaction scores (TOT_SAT), and PCMH per capita. The instrument used for collecting data was the CG-CAHPS Adult Visit 2.0 survey.

Demographics

The number of PCMH facilities was drawn from a spreadsheet prepared by the National Committee for Quality Assurance (NCQA) database administrator for each state in the U.S. (see Appendix C). The states were grouped together according to the definition of region provided by CAHPS (2013). See Table 1 below.

Table 1
Regions Throughout the U.S. According to CAHPS Definition Practice Site Characteristics

Region	States
Region 1 Northeast United States	Connecticut, Maine, Massachusetts, New Hampshire, New Jersey, New York, Pennsylvania, Puerto Rico, Rhode Island, Vermont
Region 2 Midwest United States	Illinois, Indiana, Iowa, Kansas, Michigan, Minnesota, Missouri, Nebraska, North Dakota, Ohio, South Dakota, Wisconsin
Region 3 South United States	Alabama, Arkansas, Delaware, D.C. Florida, Georgia, Kentucky, Louisiana, Maryland, Mississippi, North Carolina, Oklahoma, South Carolina, Tennessee, Texas, Virginia, West Virginia
Region 4 West United States	Alaska, Arizona, California, Colorado, Guam, Hawaii, Idaho, Montana, Nevada, New Mexico, Oregon, Utah, Washington, Wyoming

Note. Information derived from CAHPS (2014). Consumer Assessment for Healthcare Providers Survey. 2013 Chartbook: What patients say about their health care providers and medical practices.

Data Analysis

Patient satisfaction responses were examined for outliers, skewness, and kurtosis. Descriptive statistics were used to measure central tendency, measures of variability, and measures of relative standing throughout the project data. The hypothesis was assessed with a Pearson-*r* correlation coefficient. According to Ha and Ha (2012), correlation coefficient requires that the data used for a project be either interval or ratio scale. Interval variables were used to measure and analyze the correlation coefficient of patients' satisfaction scores and number of PCMH-implemented

Jacquelene S. Hamer-McGhee, DNP, MSA, RN

facilities for different regions across the U.S. Correlation coefficient measures to what extent resultant scores occupy equivalent simulated points in their distributions, meaning there is a close relationship. For instance, it is possible that lower X values to correlate with lower Y values, which is called a direct relationship or; the opposite association, where the X values associate with higher Y values (Ha & Ha, 2012).

Ha and Ha (2012) provide characteristics for correlation coefficients by noting that correlation values always have a range of strong-negative to strong- positive (-1 and +1). When the coefficient has a positive slope, this indicates an inverse relationship. If the correlation equals zero, this indicates there is no relationship at all among the variables, which supports the null hypothesis. A -1.00 coefficient implies a perfect inverse relationship among variables and a +1.00 implies a perfect direct (positive) relationship among variables.

A table for critical values of r based on degrees of freedom, N-2, was used in keeping with two constant variables that were used to measure the level of difference for both measures simultaneously. The investigator chose to use an alpha of 0.01 to find the critical value of r at the point where the null hypothesis is rejected. Rejection of the null hypothesis means r is not significantly different from zero. In the instance where the correlation coefficient was not appropriate, the non-parametric test for Spearman's rank order correlation coefficient was appropriate (Ha & Ha, 2012).

The following data contains analysis reports with a statistical description of the various measurements collected by the survey responses. The following tables and figures illustrate the gross scores assessed for each of the project variables.

Jacquelene S. Hamer-McGhee, DNP, MSA, RN

Table 2
Mean Satisfaction, PCMH Count, and PCMH by Year and Region

Year		Region				
		Midwest	Northeast	South	West	Total
2012	N	11435	5025	6312	2228	25000
	Satisfaction	0.9183	0.9194	0.9051	0.8878	0.9125
	PCMH Total	11435.00	5025.0	6312.00	2228.0	8032.61
2013	N	12118	4627	3950	4305	25000
	Satisfaction	0.9256	0.9206	0.9126	0.9117	0.9202
	PCMH Total	12118.00	4627.0	3950.0	4305.0	8095.62
Total	N	23553	9652	10262	6533	50000
	Satisfaction	0.9220	0.9200	0.9079	0.9036	0.9163
	PCMH Total	11786.40	4834.21	5402.83	3596.66	8064.12

Table 2 Illustrates that there was a slight difference in the mean scores for patient satisfaction during each year and region investigated. The number of PCMH facilities increased in the Midwest both years while the number of PCMH facilities in the Northeast decreased from 2012 to 2013. The South also saw a decline in the number of PCMH facilities from 2012 to 2013, while the Western region saw an increase.

Jacquelene S. Hamer-McGhee, DNP, MSA, RN

Table 3
Correlations: Satisfaction vs. PCMH Measures

	Satisfaction	
	R	P
PCMH total	0.049	‹ 0.001

Note. Both Pearson's correlation coefficients are extremely small; however, the values are statistically significant, due to the very large amount of data utilized.

Table 3 Illustrates the correlation for number of PCMH facilities and patient satisfaction scores overall. The p-value for PCMH total and patient satisfaction was <0.001, indicating a significance for which the null hypothesis is rejected, and the alternative is accepted (a correlation exists between the number of PCMH facilities and total patient satisfaction). However, the correlation coefficient r of 0.049 shows that there is a weak correlation between the variables.

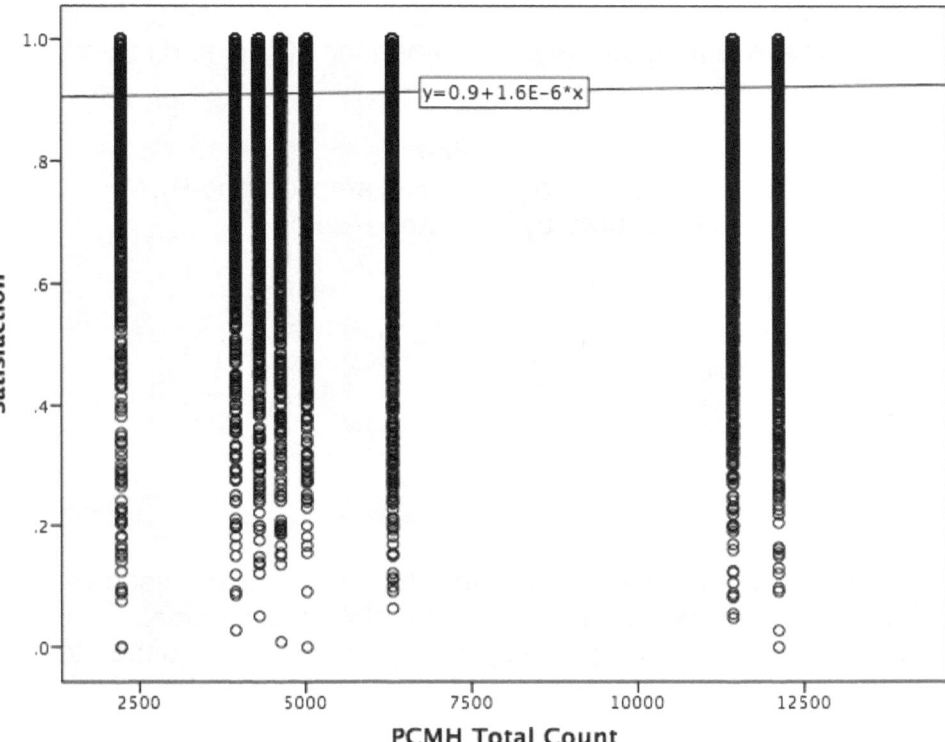

Figure 2. Scatterplot: Satisfaction vs. PCMH Total Count.

Figure 2 shows a positive relation between the variables of patient satisfaction and PCMH total (the x values are associated with higher y values). The slope line shows a + 1, which implies a perfect direct or positive relationship among the variables.

Table 4 illustrates the comparisons of mean satisfaction and PCMH total number of facilities by year and region. The satisfaction scores for year and region had *p*-values of <0.001. A statistically significant difference exists in the mean scores between year and satisfaction and region and PCMH total. The number of PCMH facilities for the year and region totals had *p*-values of 0.051 and <0.001, respectively. The *p*-value of 0.051 is not significant. There is not a statistical significance in the mean scores between the PCMH total and year. There is a statistical significance for PCMH and region.

Table 4

ANOVAs: Comparison of Mean Satisfaction and PCMH
Measures by Year and Region

	Satisfaction	*PCMH Total*
	P	P
Year	< 0.001	0.051
Region	< 0.001	< 0.001

Research Question

The research question guiding this project was based on four composites supporting patients' satisfaction. A quantitative secondary analysis approach was used to measure project data extracted from CG-CAHPS Adult Visit 2.0 survey. The project investigation focused on patients' satisfaction scores and a relationship with the number of PCMH health care facilities located in different regions of the U.S. from the years 2012 to 2013. The investigator worked to determine if there was a relationship between the number of health care facilities and overall patients' satisfaction scores in each of the four PCMH composites. The PCMH composites surveyed included timely appointments, communication with patients, courteous and helpful hospital staff; and patients' rating of the provider. The project aimed to answer the following research question:

What is the relationship between patients' satisfaction scores and the number of PCMH facilities across four regions in the U.S. from 2012 to 2013? The correlation coefficient *r* test was used to test the project hypotheses and answer the research question. Both Pearson's correlation coefficients for

Jacquelene S. Hamer-McGhee, DNP, MSA, RN

the correlation between the numbers of PCMH facilities were very small. However, the values were statistically significant due to the very large amount of data utilized. The r value of 0.049 indicated a weak correlation and the *p*-value of <0.001 indicated a statistical significance. The null hypotheses were rejected, and the alternative was accepted (There is a correlation between the number of PCMH facilities and patients' satisfaction scores).

Reliability/Validity

According to Hargraves et al. (2003), revisions for the instrument's validity and reliability have been updated and revised over time. In addition, a plan-level reliability that attains .70 for five composites occurs when there are fewer than 170 replies for each plan. Cronbach's alpha greater than or equal to .75 represents high internal consistency for two of the composites, while Cronbach's alpha ranging from .58 - .62 represents replies for items in three other composites that display less of an internal consistency (Hargraves et al., 2003).

Conclusion

The project involved a retrospective review of patient satisfaction scores and the relationship to the number of Patient Centered Medical Homes (PCMH) across the four regions for the project investigation years 2012 and 2013. The correlation coefficient tested the project hypothesis to determine whether sets of variables were related to each other. The investigator ran correlations across regions, all with the same purpose to examine if there was a significant correlation between the variables. There was no causal nature noted with the relationship, only that the variables were associated with each other. The inference is that high levels of patients' satisfaction scores were related to an increased in the number of PCMH health care facilities in certain regions of the U.S. The data were conclusive that there was statistically significant relationship between the variables. However, the correlation was weak. It should be noted that a correlation would not have been noted if a statistically significant representation of the data was not present. The weak relationship noted between patients' satisfaction scores and the number of PCMH implemented facilities was probably due to a weak design that did not have the ability to include identified PCMH and non-PCMH facilities throughout a particular state in the dataset, as identifiable PCMH facility information was not available. Further research is needed to investigate whether a PCMH-identified facility is related to increase patient satisfaction scores at the state level.

CHAPTER 5
Discussion of Findings

Introduction

The investigator provided an answer to the project research question and statistical description of the various measurements collected by the survey responses that rejected or accepted the null hypothesis. This chapter presents a series of tables and charts illustrating the gross scores assessed for each of the constructs and the interpretation of findings.

Interpretation of the Findings

The Pearson's Correlation Coefficient r test revealed that a relationship between the project's variables, patients' satisfaction scores and the number of PCMH facilities across four regions during years 2012 and 2013 was statistically significant (P-value = <0.001). The null hypothesis was rejected, and the alternative was accepted (there is a relationship between patients' satisfaction scores and the number of PCMH health care facilities in different regions in the U.S. for 2012 and 2013). See Table 3. Correlations: Satisfaction Compared to PCMH Measures. The correlation coefficient r of 0.049, shows that there is a weak correlation between the variables. According to Kellar and Kelvin (2013), large samples can yield a statistical significance even when the correlation is weak.

Hypotheses

The null and alternative hypotheses are as follows:
$H0$: There is no relationship between patients' satisfaction scores and the number of PCMH health care facilities in different regions of the U.S. for 2012 and 2013.

H1: There is a relationship between patients' satisfaction scores and the number of PCMH health care facilities in different regions of the U.S. for 2012 and 2013.

For the Pearson-r test of correlation to be valid, the following conditions must apply. Two variables must be on an interval or ratio, variables must be normally distributed and related to each other in a straight line (when two variables are graphed, they should form a straight line), and no variables can fall on the outside of the data. See Figure 2.

When determining the significance level (alpha level) for obtaining the critical value for r, an alpha of 0.01 was used. To determine the degrees of freedom (df) located on the Critical Values of the Pearson Correlation Coefficient, Appendix J, the formula n-2 (50,000 -2) was used (Kellar & Kelvin, 2013). Since the df = 49,998 and was greater than 1,000 on the critical values table, the degrees of freedom used was 1000. Using the alpha level of 0.05 and a df of 1000 from Keller and Kelvin's critical value for correlation coefficient table, the critical value equals 0.062. According to Kellar and Kelvin (2013), before a determination of whether a computed value for a correlated coefficient (r) is validated, the computed value must be greater than the critical value.

After determining the alpha level and critical value, an observation was made to ensure an independent random sample was established for all measures. There were two measures to compare; both measures were normally distributed and were of interval or ratio measurement scale, and an apparent linear relationship was present between the two variables.

Inferences about the Important Findings

Inferences and important findings from the analysis of the data addressed the project research question (What is the relationship between patients' satisfaction scores and the number of PCMH facilities across four regions in the U.S. from

Jacquelene S. Hamer-McGhee, DNP, MSA, RN

2012 to 2013?). As noted in Table 5, the data provided new information that highlighted in the descriptive statistics for each survey question. The following inferences were made about each question:

For question AV_06 (How often did patient get an appointment for urgent care as soon as needed?), 48% of sample size answered this question, N = 22,394, M = 3.55, SD = .730. The question infers that every respondent who completed the survey had an urgent appointment need. AV_06 may not have applied to every respondent. Half of the respondents skipped this question, which infers that more than half of the respondents did not have an urgent need.

The noted response rate for question AV_08 (Did patient receive appointment for non-urgent care as soon as needed?), equals 72% of the respondents who answered this question, N = 35, 802, Mean = 3.65, SD = .633. Inference is that almost three quarters of the respondents received an appointment for non-urgent care when needed.

For AV_10 (Did patient receive an answer to medical questions the same day he/she phoned provider's office?), 37% of the population answered this question, N = 18,491, Mean = 3.49, SD =.771. Inference is over one third of the respondents did receive answer to their medical questions the same day they phoned the providers office. This is a perfect example where the technology secure messaging would increase communication between the provider and patient. Providers can potentially email their patients with answers to medical questions or test results the same day, thereby increasing the patients' satisfaction with care.

Question AV_12 (Patient received an answer to medical question as soon as he/she needed when phoned provider's office after hours), 7% answered this question, N = 3,352, Mean = 3.42, SD = .885, inferring that respondents received an answer to their medical questions the same day the provider's office was called after hours. Looking at the low response to this question, one could infer that the question did not apply at the time the survey was answered. This is another opportunity to increase patient satisfaction by providing patients with answers to medical questions after hours through the nurse advice line. The nurse advise line is a 24-hour service that employs registered nurses who are specifically trained to use medical algorithms that help triage and provide advice or answers to questions patients may have. It is also tied to the secure messaging system.

Table 5
Correlations/Variables

Descriptive Statistics			
	Mean	Std. Deviation	N
AV_06	3.55	.730	22394
AV_08	3.65	.633	35802
AV_10	3.49	.771	18491
AV_12	3.42	.885	3352
AV_13	3.19	.938	48845
AV_16	1.09	.316	48712
AV_17	1.08	.311	49374
AV_19	1.10	.346	42486
AV_20	1.18	.451	49260
AV_21	1.06	.282	49475
AV_22	1.10	.350	49464
AV_25	9.22	1.364	49183
AV_27	1.11	.356	49304
AV_28	1.07	.276	49391

Table 6
Correlation Coefficient

Correlations

	AV_08	AV_10	AV_12	AV_13	AV_16	AV_17	AV_19
AV_06 Pearson Correlation	1	.672	.488	.479	.318	.238	.235	.246
Sig. (2-tailed)		.000	.000	.000	.000	.000	.000	.000
N	22394	16826	2547	22016	22016	21807	22098	20088
AV_08 Pearson Correlation	.672	1	.445	.462	.291	.225	.219	.228
Sig. (2-tailed)	.000		.000	.000	.000	.000	.000	.000
N	16826	35802	15150	2805	35400	35057	35492	31341
AV_010 Pearson Correlation	.488	.445	1	.600	.329	.308	.303	.316
Sig. (2-tailed)	000	.000		.000	.000	.000	.000	.000
N	12157	15150	18491	2805	18262	18087	18339	17137
AV_012 Pearson Correlation	.479	.462	.600	1	.321	.305	.291	.322
Sig. (2-tailed)	.000	.000	.000		.000	.000	.000	.000
N	2547	2805	2805	3352	3282	3232	48475	3135
AV_013 Pearson Correlation	.318	.291	.329	.321	1	.208	.201	.196
Sig. (2-tailed)	.000	.000	.000	.000		.000	.000	.000
N	22016	35400	18262	3282	48845	47841	48475	41737
AV_016 Pearson Correlation	.238	.225	.308	.305	.208	1	.667	.688
Sig. (2-tailed)	.000	.000	.000	.000	.000		.000	.000
N	21807	35057	18087	3232	47871	48712	48492	41724
AV_017 Pearson Correlation	.235	.219	.303	.291	.201	.667	1	.676
Sig. (2-tailed)	.000	.000	.000	.000	.000	.000		.000
N	22098	35492	18339	3304	48475	48452	45374	42251
AV_019 Pearson Correlation	.246	.228	.316	.322	.196	.688	.676	1
Sig. (2-tailed)	.000	.000	.000	.000	.000	.000	.000	
N	20088	35448	17137	3135	41737	48492	42251	42486
AV_020 Pearson Correlation	.223	.212	.274	.267	.170	.441	.478	.474
Sig. (2-tailed)	.000	.000	.000	.000	.000	.000	.000	.000
N	22064	35448	18321	3297	48363	48278	48918	42233

Jacquelene S. Hamer-McGhee, DNP, MSA, RN

AV_021 Pearson Correlation	.225	.201	.288	.272	.176	.606	.748	.625
Sig. (2-tailed)	.000	.000	.000	.000	.000	.000	.000	.000
N	22126	35356	18346	3310	48545	48449	49104	42302
AV_022 Pearson Correlation	.260	.231	.294	.309	.227	.570	.633	.568
Sig. (2-tailed)	.000	.000	.000	.000	.000	.000	.000	.000
N	22111	35530	18331	3299	48526	48451	49096	42271
AV_025 Pearson Correlation	.328	.305	.400	.377	.273	.574	.618	.595
Sig. (2-tailed)	.000	.000	.000	.000	.000	.000	.000	.000
N	22001	35337	18213	3274	48253	48151	48770	41999
AV_027 Pearson Correlation	.262	.236	.290	.263	.206	.197	.194	.191
Sig. (2-tailed)	.000	.000	.000	.000	.000	.000	.000	.000
N	22047	35397	18265	3279	48352	48267	48905	42104
. AV_028 Pearson Correlation	.214	.194	.230	.231	.176	.182	.192	.173
Sig. (2-tailed)	.000	.000	.000	.000	.000	.000	.000	.000
N	22083	35466	18318	3295	48435	48350	48984	42189

** Correlation is significant at the 0.01 level (2-tailed).

Correlations

	AV_20	AV_21	AV_22	AV_25	AV_27	AV_28
AV_022 Pearson Correlation	.428	.618	1	.566	.206	.198
Sig. (2-tailed)	.000	.000		.000	.000	.000
N	49026	49261	49464	48917	49044	49120
AV_025 Pearson Correlation	.522	.615	.566	1	.243	.216
Sig. (2-tailed)	.000	.000	.000		.000	.000
N	48699	48924	48917	49183	48754	48828
AV_027 Pearson Correlation	.197	.185	.206	.243	1	.712
Sig. (2-tailed)	.000	.000	.000	.000		.000
N	48819	49056	49044	48754	49304	49069
AV_028 Pearson Correlation	.175	.194	.198	.216	.712	1
Sig. (2-tailed)	.000	.000	.000	.000	.000	
N	48899	49135	49120	48828	49069	49391

Jacquelene S. Hamer-McGhee, DNP, MSA, RN

Note. Correlation is significant at the 0.01 level (2-tailed). The correlation tables consist of a 14 x 14 table that has 200 items. The number of items increases to 800 when the four regions are included (NE, MW, S, and W). Weak to strong correlations were noted throughout the correlation tables. The strongest and weakest correlations are discussed in Chapter 5 analysis.

Based on the population investigated, the strongest correlation occurred between survey questions AV_21 (Provider showed respect for what patient had to say) and AV_17 (Provider listened carefully to patient): .748. Overall this pair of survey questions appeared to reveal positive provider communication with the patient. Frequency tables support the positive communication responses. Ninety-two percent answered yes to question AV_17 and 1.09% answered no. Responses for AV_21 were 93.61% answered yes and 0.98 % answered no.

The correlation between question AV_27 (Were clerks and receptionists helpful?) and question AV_28 (Were clerks and receptionists courteous and respectful?) also revealed a strong correlation: .712. Overall, these survey questions were both related to staff communication. The weakest correlation, .170, occurred between questions AV_20 (Did provider know the important information about patient's medical history?) and AV_13 (Did patient see their provider within 15 minutes of appointment time?). Both questions were provider focused, but they are not closely related. The frequency table for question AV_20 reported that 83.16 responded with yes, while 12.73 said yes, somewhat, 1.27 did not respond and 2.83 said no. Question AV_13 reported that 1.99% did not respond, 8.62 said never, 32.52 said usually, and 45.21 said always. With this pair of questions, patients appeared to be satisfied with their care over half of the time for provider knowledge and less than half of the time for seeing their provider in 15 minutes or less.

Questions 6-12 strongly related versus question 13, which was a weak relation. Statistical significance noted for 6-12 vs. question 16, which had a weak to medium relationship. For question 25, an overall provider satisfaction question, related weakly to access survey questions but were strongly related to communication survey question. See Table 7 below for survey questions grouped into constructs.

Table 7
Pearson-r Correlated Coefficient Scores from Paired Survey Questions

Question	Score
AV_21 During your most recent visit did this provider seem to know the important information about your medical history?	
AV_17 During your most recent visit did this provider listen carefully to you?	.748 - Strongest
AV_27 During your most recent visit, were clerks' receptions at this provider's office as helpful as you thought they should be?	
AV_28 During your most recent visit did clerks and receptionists at this provider's office treat you with courtesy and respect?	.712 - Strong
AV_20 During your most recent visit did this provider seem to know the important information about your medical history?	
AV_13 Wait time includes time spent in the waiting room and exam room. In the last 12 months, how often did you see this provider within 15 minutes of your appointment time?	.170 - Weak

Table 8

CG-CAHPS Adult 2.0 Survey Composites and Corresponding Questions

Clinician and Group CAHPS Adult 2.0 Survey	*Survey Questions*
Getting Timely Appointments, Care, and Information	AV_6 In the last 12 months, when you phoned this provider's office to get an appointment you needed right away, how often did you get an appointment as soon as possible?
	AV_8 In the last 12 months, when did you make an appointment for a check-up or routine care with this provider, how often did you get an appointment as soon as you needed?
	AV_10 In the last 12 months, when you phoned this provider's office during regular office hours, how often did you get an answer to your medical question the same day?
	AV_12 In the last 12 months, when you phoned this provider's office after regular office hours, how often did you get an answer to your medical question as soon as you needed?
	AV_13 Wait time includes time spent in the waiting room and exam room. In the last 12 months, how often did you see this provider within 15 minutes of your appointment time?
How Well Providers Communicate with Patients	AV_16 During your most recent visit, did this provider explain things in a way that was easy to understand?
	AV_17 During your most recent visit did this provider listen carefully to you?
	AV_19 During your most recent visit, did this provider give you easy to understand information about these health questions or concerns?
	AV_20 During your most recent visit did this provider seem to know the important information about your medical history?
	AV_21 During your most recent visit did this provider seem to know the important information about your medical history?
	AV_22 During your most recent visit, did this provider spend enough time with you?

Helpful, Courteous, and Respectful Office Staff	AV_27 During your most recent visit, were clerks' receptions at this provider's office as helpful as you thought they should be?
	AV_28 During your most recent visit, did clerks and receptionists at this provider's office treat you with courtesy and respect?
Patient's Rating of the Provider	AV_25 Using any number from 0-10, where 0 is the worst provider possible and 10 is the best provider possible, what number would you use to rate this provider?

Note. Information derived from CAHPS, (2014). Consumer Assessment for Healthcare Providers Survey. 2013 Chart book: What patients say about their health care providers and medical practices.

Implications of Analysis for Leaders

After answering the research question, interpreting the findings, and highlighting the inferences of those findings, the investigator found there is an opportunity for robust knowledge sharing. Descriptive statistics revealed that patients appeared to be very concerned about communication with their health care provider. Implications for leadership are consistent with information discussed in the project literature where Brennan and Monson (2014) focused on discovering qualities and responsibilities that raise an organizational team-based culture of professionalism.

Therefore, strong implications for health care leaders to develop programs that will provide communication training for employees that will promote and sustain good communication with their patients. Good communication is believed to encourage patients to be involved in the maintenance of their care. Patients expect everyone on their health care team to function as a unit to deliver the best possible care.

Through the analysis of patient satisfaction data, nurse leaders and other health care executives may develop a heightened awareness of patient concerns and identify

Jacquelene S. Hamer-McGhee, DNP, MSA, RN

existing gaps in care that are not patient focused. Identifying the gaps in patient focused care may also lend to informed decision about processes and resources that increase patients' satisfaction for the overall patient experience. Gaps in the patients' satisfaction data may be especially important where there is a particularly weak or strong correlation between patient satisfaction and provider/staff inter-professionalism. As mentioned in the project literature review, patients tend to trust that each member of the team is expertly trained to perform their specific job (McLaughlin & Kaluzny, 2006). Brennan and Monson (2014) mentioned how important it is to strategize positive values and inter-professional relationships through alignment of organizational systems and structures.

The World Health Organization (WHO) reports that patient engagement allows the patient to learn more about their diagnosis and treatment care-plan. Evidence proves that when patients are engaged and informed about their care, anxiety decreases and fosters patient satisfaction. When a patient is not anxious about their care, they will pay more attention to the recommendations made by their health by their provider and make informed decisions about how to maintain their health. Satisfied and engaged patients are less likely to visit the emergency department (ED) for routine primary care or be readmitted to the hospital in less than 30 days.

Recommendations

The investigator analyzed data relationships between related patients' responses based on the four project composites: Access to health care, communication, courteous staff, and provider scoring, which revealed new and potentially important information for what patients are reporting about their health care providers and staff. Through the analysis of patient satisfaction data, nurse leaders and other health care executives may develop a heightened awareness of patient concerns and identify existing gaps in care that are not patient focused. Identifying the gaps in patient focused care may also lend to informed decision about processes and resources that increase patients' satisfaction the overall patient experience. Gaps in the patients' satisfaction data may be especially important where there is a particularly weak or strong correlation between the project variables.

Recommendations for improving and increasing patient satisfaction begin with executive leadership acknowledgement and endorsement of patient satisfaction and patient experience of care priorities within the organization's strategic goals. The organization must be on board with what the process is for improve identified issues, barriers and gaps to patient centered care. All employees of an organization need to understand the importance and benefits of communicating with the patient and among each other.

Recommendations for Future Research

Past methods and strategies for maintaining a robust health care organization have slowly trickled away while new mandates have rapidly moved in. Health care leaders are now expected to take what is left and function with new technology, innovation, and culture changes for today's consumers of care. To meet this challenge, realignment of health care systems' structure and outdated clinical processes must take effect in organizations to accommodate chronic care management as an essential health care goal of the PCMH model (Carlstrom & Ekman, 2012).

Accomplishing high levels of patient satisfaction involves hospital management acceptance and participation in patient-centered care progress initiatives. Hospital leadership is also expected to engage frontline clinicians in this process

(Rozenblum et al., 2013). However, additional investigation is necessary to determine to what degree new primary care models, such as PCMH, affect patient satisfaction, patient health care outcomes, improved access to care between variations of practice types, and increased patient engagement (Paustian et al., 2013).

An increase in the enhanced primary care concept is supported by research to improve patient experiences, their health care outcomes, and satisfaction with their care (IOM, 2012; Naylor & Kurtzman, 2010). Nevertheless, research for increasing the PCMH concept and its relationship to patients' satisfaction and experience of care has only scratched the surface for what lies ahead in health care. Analysis for the data reported in this project supported that an increase in the number of available PCMH facilities, potentially increases the number of patients who will have access to health care.

Conversely, since PCMH effectiveness is difficult to measure without narrowing the scope to identifying specific health care facilities or if the PCMH model is attributed to increased patient satisfaction scores at the regional level, more research is needed at the state level. Research at the state level to determine if there is a significant difference in mean scores before and after PCMH implementation, could potentially be helpful to health care executives on how best to allocate resources for developing and sustaining PCMH strategies. A limitation for the project design presented because the ability to determine if the facilities that reported to the CAHPS database were PCMH or non-PCMH facilities was not an option available at this time.

Summary

The purpose of this quantitative non-experimental project was to determine if there is a relationship between the overall patient satisfaction CAHPS scores and the number of PCMH facilities by regions in the United States for calendar years 2012 and 2013. The investigator was able to report a relationship between variables in the data by using the Pearson-r Correlation Coefficient test.

The problem addressed was health care administrators and leaders tend to overlook how implementing PCMH affects patients' satisfaction scores despite the evidence to support improving quality in the primary health care environments. According to Rozenblum et al., (2013) and Becker (2013), health care providers and administrators also struggle to acknowledge that poor customer service, lack of patient-centered care, and the lack of patient engagement are the most likely causes of poor patients' satisfaction scores (Becker, 2013).

Leaders in the health care community exhibit strong opinions about care coordination, patient self-management, and improved access to care as the top priorities for PCMH (Wexler et al., 2012). More work is needed in the U.S. to adequately process and implement standards designed to measure and improve patients' satisfaction and quality of care through the implementation of patient-centered care and the PCMH model of care.

The literature review revealed studies focused on developing actionable conceptual frameworks for patient-centered care (Green, 2012; Hobbs, 2009; Lusk & Fater, 2013). Methods used for the studies throughout the literature review included quantitative, quantitative, descriptive analysis, conceptualization, case project methodology, exploratory, explanatory, and descriptive. Other pilot studies uncovered statistical significance for the implementation of PCMH using frameworks, such as Donabedian and IOM. The theoretical framework used to guide this project was the Donabedian's health care quality framework.

There was no causal nature noted with the relationship of project variables, only that the variables were associated with each other. The inference is that high levels of patients' satisfaction scores were related to and increased the number of health care facilities in certain regions of the U.S. The data were conclusive that there was statistically significant relationship between the variables. Further research is needed to investigate whether a PCMH-identified facility before and after implementation is related to increase patient satisfaction scores at the state level.

References

Administration on Aging. (2014, September 29). U.S. Department of Health and Human Services: Administration for Community Living. Retrieved from http://www.aoa.gov/AoARoot/Aging_Statistics/future_growth/aging21/demography.aspx

Agency for Healthcare Research and Quality. (2006). *The High Concentration of U.S. Health Care Expenditures.* Rockville, MD: Agency for Healthcare Research and Quality.

Agency for Healthcare Research and Quality. (2014). *The CAHPS Clinician & Group Survey Database.* Retrieved from http://www.ahrq.gov

Alexander, J., & Bae, D. (2012). Does the patient-centered medical home work? A critical synthesis of research on patient-centered medical homes and patient-related outcomes. *Health Services Management Research, 25(2),*51-59. doi: 10.1258/hsmr.2012.012001

Berwick, D. (2002). A user's manual for the IOM's Quality Chasm Report. *Health Affairs , 21*(3), 80-90.

Bleich, S., Osaltin, E., & Murray, C. (2009). How does satisfaction with the health-care system relate to patient experience? *Bulletin of the World Health Organization, 87* (4), 271-278. doi: 10.2471/bit.07.050401

Bottone, F., Musich, S., & Wang, S. (2014). Obese older adults report high satisfaction and positive experiences. *BMC Health Services Research, 14* (1), 1-10. doi: 10.1186/1472-6963-14-220

Brennan, M., & Monson, V. (2014). Professionalism: Good for patients and health care organizations. *Mayo Clinical Proceedings,89* (5), 646-652.doi: 10.1016/jimayocp.2014.01.011

Carlstrom, E., & Ekman, I. (2012). Organizational culture and change: Implementing person-centered care. *Journal of Health Organization and Management, 26*(2), 175-191. doi:10.1108/14777261211230763

Consumer Assessment Healthcare Providers and Systems. (2014). *The Clinician & Group Survey Database: Practice site characteristics.* Retrieved from www.cahpsdatabase.ahrq.gov.

Centers for Medicare & Medicaid Services (CMS). (2014). Centers for Medicare and Medicaid Services Retrieved from http://www.cms.gov/site-search/search-results.html?q=medicare%20advantage%20cms

Cromwell, J., Trisolini, M., Pope, G., Mitchell, J., & Greenwald, L. (2011). *Pay for performance in health care: Methods and approaches.* doi.10.378/rti.2011.bk.0002.1103. Research Triangle Park, NC: RTI Press publication.

Detsky, J., & Shaul, R. (2013). Incentives to increase patient satisfaction: Are we doing more harm than good? *Canadian Medical Association Journal , 185*(14), 1199-1200.doi: 10.1503/cmaj.13036

Egger, M., Day, J., Scammon, D. Y., Wilson, A., & Magill, M. (2012). Correlation of the care by design primary care practice redesign model and the priniciples of the patient-centered medical home. *JABFM , 25* (2), 216-223. doi: 10.3122/jabfm.2012.02.110159

Furlow, B. (2014). Engaged, informed patients help ensure better outcomes. Retrieved from http://www.empr.com/engaged-informed-patients-help-ensure-better-outcomes/article/368984/

Greene, S., Tuzzio, L., & Cherkin, D. (2012). A framework for making patient-centered care front and center. *The Permanente, 16* (3), 49-53.

Ha, R., & Ha, J. (2012). *Integrative statistics for the social and behavior.* Thousand Oaks, CA: Sage.

Hargraves, J., Hays, R., & Cleary, P. (2003). Psychometric properties of the consumer assessment health plans study. *Health Service Research*, 1509-1528. doi:10.1111/j.1475-6773.2003.00190.x

Hibbard, J., & Green, J. (2013). What evidence shows about patient activation: better health outcomes and care experiences. *Health Affairs*, *32*(2), 2207-214. doi:10.1377/hlthaff.2012.1061

Hobbs, J. (2009). A dimensional analysis of patient-centered care. *Nursing Research*, 52-59.

Instituted of Medicine. (2011). *Engineering a learning healthcare system: A look at the future: Workshop summary.* Washington, DC: The National Academies Press.

Institute of Medicine. (2012). Implementing the institute of medicine future of nursing report-part III: How nurses are solving some of primary care's most pressing challenges. *IOM Report*, 1-8.

Kellar, S., & Kelvin, E. (2013). *Munro's statistical methods for healthcare research* (6th ed.). Philadelphia, PA: Wolters Kluwer Health/Lippincott Williams & Wilkins.

Langford, R. (2001). *Navigating the Maze of Nursing Research.* St. Louis, MO: Mosby.

Lusk, M., & Fater, K. (2013). A concept analysis of patient-centered care. *Nursing Forum , 48*(2), 89-98. doi: 10.1111/nug.12019

McHugh, M., Arnold, J., & Buschman, P. (2012). Nurses leading the response to the crisis of palliative care for vulnerable populations. *Nursing Economics, 30*(3), 140-147.

McLaughlin, P., & Kaluzny, A. (2006). *Continuous quality improvement* (3rd ed.). Sudbury, MA: Jones & Bartlett.

Morrison, E. (2011). *Ethics in health admininistratrion: A practical approach for decision makers* (2nd ed.). Sudbury, MA: Jones and Bartlett.

Naylor, M., & Kurtzman, E. (2010). The role of nurse practitioners in reinventing primary care. *Health Affairs, 29*(5), 893-899. doi:10.1377/hlthaff.2010.0440

Jacquelene S. Hamer-McGhee, DNP, MSA, RN

Nelson, K., Helfrich, C., Sun, H., Hebert, P., Liu, C., Dolan, E...Fihn, S. (2014). Implementation of the paient-centered medical home in the veterans health administration: Associations with patient satisfaction, quality of care, staff burnout, and hospital and emergency department use. *JAMA Internal Medicine, 174*(8), 1350-1358. doi: 10.1001/jamainternmed.2014.2488

Nielsen, M. (2014, February 12). PCPCC supports SGR repeal and Medicare Provider Payment Modernization Act. Patient Centered Primary Care Collaborative. Retrieved from http://edit.pcpcc.net/2014/02/12/pcpcc-supports-sgr-repeal-and-medicare-provider-payment-modernization-act

Oldenburg, J., Chase, D., Christensen, K., & Trittle, B. (2013). *Engage!: Transforming healthcare through digital patient engagement.* Chicago, IL: Health Information and Management Systems Society (HIMSS).

Patel, M., Arron, M., Sinsky, T., Green, E., Baker, D., Bowen, J., et al. (2013). Estimating the Staffing Infrastructure for PCMH. *The American Journal of Managed Care , 19(6)*, 509-515.

Paustian, M. L., Alexander, J. A., Reda, D. K., Wise, C. G., Green, L. A., & Fetters, M. D. (2013). Partial and incremental PCMH practice transformation: Implications for quality costs. *Health Services Research*, 49(1), 1-18.doi: 10.1111/1475-6773.12085

Primary Care Collaborative. (2009). *Proof in practice: A compilation of patient-centered medical home pilot and demonstration projects.* Washington, DC: Patient-Centered Primary Care Collaborative.

Ramano, P., Hussey, P., & Ritley, D. (2010). *Selecting quality and resource use measures: A decision guide for community quality collaboratives.* Rockville, MD: Agency for Healthcare Research and Quality.

Reinerstsen, J., Gosfield, A., Rupp, W., & Whittington, J. (2007). Engaging physicians in a shared quality agenda. *Institute for Healthcare Improvement*, 1-46.

Resources, T. D. (2014, 5 11). About the law. Retrieved from http://www.hhs.gov/healthcare/rights/index.html#PAGE_2

Robinson, J., Callister, L., Berry, A., & Dearing, K. (2008). Patient-centered care and adherence: Definitions and applications to improve outcomes. *Journal of the American Academy of Nurse Practitioners, 20*(12), 600-607. doi:10.1111/j.1745-7599.2008.00360.x

Rosland, A., Nelson, K., Sun, H., Dolan, E., Maynard, C., Bryson, C., et al. (2012). The patient-centered medical home in the Veterans Health Administration. *The American journal of managed care , 19(7)*, e263-72.

Rozenblum, R., Lisby, M., Hockey, P., Levtzion-Korach, O., Salzberg, C., Efrati, N., et al. (2013). The patient satisfaction chasm: The gap between hospital management and frontline clinicians. *BMJ Quality and Saftey*, 242-250.

Schwenk, T. (2014). The patient-centered medical home: One size does not fit all. *JAMA , 311*(8), 802-803. doi:10.1001/jama.2014.352

Sharma, A. (2012). What is ex-post facto research? Explain? Retrieved from http://www.
preservearticles.com/2012030825859/what-is-ex-post-facto-research-explain. Html

Spooner, B., Reese, B., & Konschak, C. (2012). *Accountable care: Bridging the health information technology divide.* Viginia Beach, VA: Convergent.

Tremblay, D., Touati, N., Roberge, D., Denis, J., Turcotte, A., & Samson, B. (2014). Conditions for production of interdisciplinary teamwork outcomes in oncology teams: Protocol for a realist evaluation. *Implementation Science, 9*(1), 11. doi:10.1186/1748-5908-9-76

Wexler, R., King, D., & Andrews, M. (2012). Comparison of patient and physician opinion of patient centered medical home fundamentals. *Southern Medical Journal, 105*(4), 238.

Appendix A

Patient-Centered Medical Home Principles and Overview Data adapted from Patient Centered Primary Care Collaborative (2009)

Patient Centered Medical Home (PCMH) Principals	Strategies for Implementations	Examples of Specific Components	Staffing Requirements
1. Provider Directed Patient Centered Care	Care Management Behavioral Health Social Problems Population Health, TeamSTEPPS	Management of patient before, intra, and post, health care encounter Depression, Suicidal, Anxiety, Coping, resources to manage health status Manage a population of patients (i.e., Chronic Diseases Diabetes, HTN), HEDIS Nutrition Care Spiritual Care	Phys., RN, PA, LPN, NA Nurse Case Management Behavioral Health Specialist Social Worker Registered Dietician Registered Dietician Clergy
2. Patient Safety and Quality	Medication Management Data Analysis	Medication Reconciliation, Pain Control, Pain Contracts Clinical Practice Guidelines	Pharmacist, Data Clinical Practice Manager

Jacquelene S. Hamer-McGhee, DNP, MSA, RN

3. Coordinated and Integrated Care 4. Physician Continuity	Patient information is accessible to all health care providers across the health care continuum Automated Health Records, Comprehensive Care plan	Referrals to specialty providers, diagnostics tests and procedures, lab values, images and artifacts, Patient encounters occur with the same provider each visit, or someone on their PCMH team	PCMH Team Clinical Practice Managers,
5. Access to Care (ATC)	Decrease ATC barriers, non-emergent ED visits, readmissions < 30 days, Adequate staffing for patient load	Adequate availability of appointments, Template management, Secure Messaging, Mobile devices and applications, personal health information, Health care info Tele-health, language needs, Nurse advice line, Community care, Robust Dashboards	RN, Linguist program, Heath Information Technology (HIT)
6. Pay for Performance	Patient satisfaction metrics, patient health care outcomes Coding and billing accuracy, upgraded coding system	Engaged patients and staff, Patient-centered culture ICD-10 implementation	Patient, PCMH Team, Coding personnel, HIT personnel

Note. **Phys**-Physician, **PA**-Physician Assistant, **RN**-Registered Nurse, **LPN**-Licensed Practical Nurse, **NA**-Nursing Assistant, **HTN**-Hypertension, **HEDIS**-, Healthcare Effectiveness Data and Information Set, **TeamSTEPPS**- Team Strategies & Tools to

Jacquelene S. Hamer-McGhee, DNP, MSA, RN

Enhance Performance & Patient Safety , HIT-Health Information Technology, ED-Emergency Department, ICD-10-International Statistical Classification of Diseases and Related Health Problems, 10th Revision.

Appendix B

CAHPS® Clinician & Group Surveys

Version: Visit Survey 2.0

Population: Adult

Language: English

Notes

- **Time referent:** The Visit Survey asks respondents about experiences during their most recent visit with a provider, as opposed to all their visits with that provider in the last 12 months. However, most questions about access to care refer to experiences over the last 12 months.

- **References to "this provider" rather than "this doctor:"** This survey uses "this provider" to refer to the individual specifically named in Question 1. A "provider" could be a doctor, nurse practitioner, physician assistant, or other individual who provides clinical care. Survey users may change "provider" to "doctor" throughout the questionnaire. For guidance, please see **Preparing a Questionnaire Using the CAHPS Clinician & Group Surveys.**

- **Supplemental items:** CAHPS supplemental items for this survey are currently in development. In the meantime, users can adapt some supplemental items developed for the 12-Month Survey that are available in the **Clinician & Group Surveys and Instructions.** For assistance, please contact the CAHPS Help Line at cahps1@ahrq.gov or 1-800-492-9261.

Jacquelene S. Hamer-McGhee, DNP, MSA, RN

- **Assessing domains of the Patient-Centered Medical Home (PCMH):** To evaluate the domains of a medical home, survey users are encouraged to use the CAHPS Clinician & Group 12-Month Survey with the Patient-Centered Medical Home items rather than the Visit Survey. A pre-assembled survey that combines the 12-Month Survey with the PCMH supplemental items is available in the **Clinician & Group Surveys and Instructions.**

Documents Available for the CAHPS Clinician & Group Surveys

This document is part of a comprehensive set of instructional materials that address implementing the Clinician & Group Surveys, analyzing the data, and reporting the results. All documents are available on the Agency for Healthcare Research and Quality's Web site: www.cahps.ahrq.gov. For assistance in accessing these documents, please contact the CAHPS Help Line at 800-492-9261 or cahps1@westat.com.

For descriptions of these documents, refer to: **What's Available for the Clinician & Group Survey**

Questionnaires

CAHPS Clinician & Group Surveys: Overview of the Questionnaires

- **12-Month Survey 2.0** (Adult and Child, English and Spanish)
- **Patient-Centered Medical Home Survey** (Adult and Child, English and Spanish)
- **Visit Survey 2.0** (Adult and Child, English and Spanish)

Supplemental Items

- **Supplemental Items for the Adult Surveys**
- **Supplemental Items for Child Surveys**

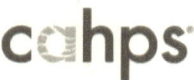

Jacquelene S. Hamer-McGhee, DNP, MSA, RN

- About the Item Set for Addressing Health Literacy
- About the Cultural Competence Item Set
- About the Health Information Technology Item Set
- About the Patient-Centered Medical Home (PCMH) Item Set

Survey Administration Guidelines

- Preparing a Questionnaire Using the CAHPS Clinician & Group Surveys
- Fielding the CAHPS Clinician & Group Surveys
- Sample Notification Letters for the CAHPS Clinician & Group Surveys
- Sample Telephone Script for the CAHPS Clinician & Group Surveys
- Guidelines for Translating CAHPS Surveys

Data Analysis Program and Guidelines

- CAHPS Analysis Program (SAS)
- Preparing and Analyzing Data from the CAHPS Clinician & Group Surveys
- Instructions for Analyzing Data from CAHPS Surveys

Reporting Measures and Guidelines

- Patient Experience Measures for the CAHPS Clinician & Group Surveys

Appendix C

State	Diabetes Recognition Program	Heart/Stroke Recognition Program	Physician Practice Connection		Patient Centered Medical Home (PPC-PCMH & PCMH)				
	Clincians	Clincians	Clinicians	Sites	Clincians	Sites	Level 1	Level 2	Level 3
Miltary OCONUS					67	25	0	4	21
AK	5				100	4	0	1	3
AL	151	31			166	37	11	13	13
AR	14	25			181	58	0	9	49
AZ	102	175			283	65	1	17	47
CA	1444	809			2428	241	15	50	176
CO	400	237	4	1	1138	161	6	21	134
CT	80	102			757	196	12	20	164
DC	34				100	17	0	2	15
DE					45	10	2	5	3
FL	319	268	1	1	1063	333	33	53	247
GA	204	92			692	153	14	13	126
HI					341	57	12	8	37
IA	63	27			381	60	0	28	32
ID					119	21	0	3	18
IL	396	238			992	245	20	24	201
IN	218	19			248	50	2	16	32
KS	48	2			268	60	0	5	55
KY	113				318	73	9	14	50
LA	94	47			373	85	26	21	38
MA	75				1548	174	22	20	132
MD	153	3			607	125	7	25	93
ME	440	427	87	27	755	173	10	58	105
MI	122	7			393	136	24	23	89
MN	1				174	6	1	1	4
MO	276	100			680	158	8	9	141
MS	55	5			64	27	3	19	5
MT	22				179	35	5	18	12
NC	902	482	237	45	2062	491	31	37	423
ND					9	2	0	2	0
NE	92	40			143	23	0	1	22
NH	64	6			383	60	2	14	44
NJ	51	1			669	170	12	25	133
NM	1				273	37	13	10	14
NV			3	1	172	60	0	3	47
NY	2048	145	55	8	5542	1045	117	76	852
OH	553	85			1231	334	39	47	248
OK	18	7			167	12	1	3	8
OR	63				395	32	6	1	25
PA	263	62	2	1	2260	468	106	61	301
PR					62	9	3	6	0
RI					319	79	10	3	66
SC	256	155			422	97	7	10	80
SD					4	2	0	0	2
TN	192	159			542	111	9	19	83
TX	385	272	22	5	1585	335	21	48	266
UT					10	4	0	2	2
VA	239	105			693	166	3	8	156
VT	1				570	120	11	40	69
WA	276	22			1236	116	6	23	87
WI	489	33			1103	178	2	17	159
WV	1				169	32	12	7	13
WY	5				11	4	1	1	2
Total	10728	4188	411	89	34492	6762	655	964	5143

Recognition Programs: Number of Clinicians and Sites Recognized as of (12/31/2013)

Jacquelene S. Hamer-McGhee, DNP, MSA, RN

Appendix D

Visit Survey Adult 2.0

These instructions and accompanying data file layout specifications apply to the:

CAHPS Clinician & Group Data File Specifications

Submitting data to the CAHPS Database requires survey data to be organized by group, practice site and provider in order to receive access to the CAHPS Database Online Reporting System.

Number of files to be submitted

Three separate flat files (Group Data File, Practice Site Data File and Sample Data File) make up a CG-CAHPS submission and are detailed in this document.

Group Data File: Each line in the group data file represents a medical group. Multiple groups can be added to the data file using unique IDs for each.

A group can be defined as a medical group, ACO, state organization or some other grouping of practice sites. A group is not a vendor organization.

The **Group ID** variable must be consistent to link the group, practice site and the sample files.

The **Group Name** variable is exactly how the name will be displayed in the Online Reporting System.

The **Group Contact Name, Phone and Email** are required at the group level to receive access to reporting. Do not provide vendor information.

Practice Site Data File: Each line in the practice site data file represents a practice site. Multiple practice sites can be added to the data file using unique IDs for each practice site and matching IDs to the related group.

A practice site can be considered a medical office. A practice site is an outpatient facility in a specific location. Each practice site located in a building containing multiple medical offices is considered a separate practice site. Providers in a single practice site should share administrative and clinical support staff.

Jacquelene S. Hamer-McGhee, DNP, MSA, RN

The **Practice Site ID** variable must be consistent to link the group, practice site and the sample files.

The **Practice Site Name** variable is exactly how the name will be displayed in the Online Reporting System.

The **Practice Site Contact Name, Phone and Email** are required at the group level to receive access to reporting. Do not provide vendor information.

Sample Data File: Each line in the sample data file represents a sampled individual.

A record must be submitted for each sampled individual. For unreturned surveys, leave all question fields blank.

Visit Survey Adult 2.0
Data files are associated through IDs

Each of the required data files includes one or more ID fields. These ID fields (and their associated values) are critically important as they create a link between the data files that are submitted. For example, the Sample data file specification requires that each record include not only a unique "person-level" identification number, but each person-level record must also include an ID field that represents each of the Groups and Practice Sites that were surveyed.

The following example illustrates how the Group data file, Practice Site data file, and Sample data files are related to one another via the ID fields when there is more than one Group.

This example shows that there are two (2) Groups (Preferred Medical System and Health America Group). The Group ID numbers for these two Groups are repeated in both the Sample data file and in the Practice Site data file. This example also shows that practice sites Oak Street Clinic and Elm Street Clinic are affiliated with the Preferred Medical System (Group ID =2222222221 for Practice Site ID 100000001 and for Practice Site ID 10000000).

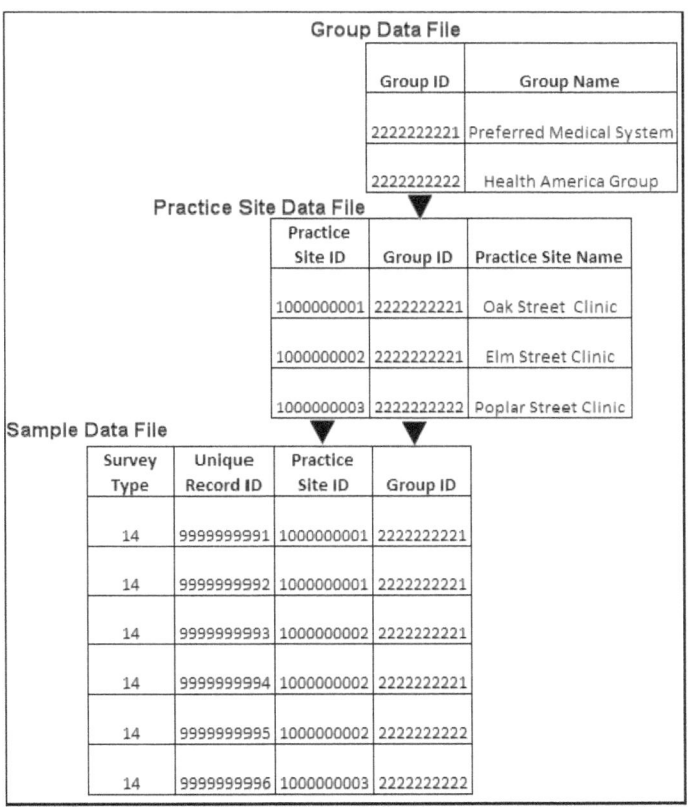

Example 1: Associated Group and Practice Site IDs

Visit Survey Adult 2.0

Reporting structure

The structure of the files and the IDs used for linking the three files reflects how the data will be reported. Using the previous example, two Group reports and three Practice Site reports would be generated. The Group Contact would have access to Group and Practice Site reporting, while the Practice Site contact can only access the individual Practice Site reports. Here are how the reports would look: Preferred Medical System (aggregated results of Oak and Elm Street Clinics)

- Oak Street Clinic
- Elm Street Clinic

- Health America Group (same results for both the group and practice site)
- Poplar Street Clinic

Additional information about the data files

Group Data File. The Group data file contains one record for each unique Group that participated in the survey and describes the "parent" organization(s).

Practice sites are considered to be "children" of the parent organization and are defined in the Practice Site data file. Practice Sites that are not a part of a parent organization are NOT required to submit a Group data file. However, they must submit a Practice Site and Sample data file.

Each Group must be uniquely numbered using the Group ID field. There is a 50- character Group Name field that is used to name each Group in the reporting.

Practice Site Data File. The Practice Site data file contains one record for each unique practice site that participated in the survey. Each practice site must be uniquely numbered using the "Practice Site ID" field. There is a 50-character field that is used to name each practice site (practice site name).

If the practice sites are named similarly, consider using as many of the 50 characters as necessary to distinguish among them. For example, "Primary Care Health Clinic – West" or "Primary Care Health Clinic – East".

Sample Data File. The Sample data file contains ID fields that are associated with the Group file and with the Practice Site file. Make certain that the values assigned to these ID fields are in agreement with the corresponding ID fields and values in the other file(s).

Each record in the Sample data file must be uniquely numbered using the field "Unique Record ID". This file must contain **one record for every person who was sampled** to participate in the survey – irrespective of the final disposition or survey status (e.g., completed survey, ineligible, refused to participate, etc.) The file specifications provide detailed information about the values that can be assigned for survey disposition.

Visit Survey Adult 2.0

File format. All data files are to be submitted in flat, ASCII file format and must conform to the file layout specifications.

As noted above, it is critical that the values assigned for the ID fields accurately correspond to one another.

Jacquelene S. Hamer-McGhee, DNP, MSA, RN

ID fields in the Sample, Practice Site, and Group data files are 10 digits in length. DO NOT assign any ID values with a leading "0" (zero).

Missing Value Assignments

Make sure to use double digit missing values for questions with 2 field positions.

Reason for missing value	Application	Missing value
Appropriately skipped	Indicates the respondent appropriately skipped this question.	7 or 77
Multiple mark	Multiple marks made it impossible to identify the response.	8 or 88
Missing	No response, not part of skip pattern.	9 or 99
Question not included	A question is not included in the survey questionnaire.	Blank

Group File Layout

Visit Survey Adult 2.0

- Group data file must be in ascii/flat format.
- The file must contain one record for each Group that administered the survey.

Jacquelene S. Hamer-McGhee, DNP, MSA, RN

- Group ID in this file must match IDs in Practice Site and Sample data files.
- The data file must conform to the layout specifications below.

Variable Description	Field Position	Value Labels	Details/Comments
Group ID	1-10	10 characters	Unique ID used to match records in this Group data file to the Sample Level data file & Practice Site data file
Group Name	11-60	50 characters	Name of the group. Use unique names to distinguish entities for reporting purpose. This is the name that will appear in the Online Reporting System.
Street	61-90	30	
Street	91-120	30	Floor or Suite
City	121-150	30	
State	151-152	2 character	2-character state abbreviation (e.g., AL)
Zip Code	153-157	XXXXX	5-digit zip code
Phone Number	158-167	XXXXXX XXXX	10-digit telephone number. (*do not include spaces or dashes.*)
Group Ownership and Affiliation	168-169	01 = Provider(s) and/or Physician(s) 02 = Hospital or Health	Ownership or affiliation type that best describes this group.
Group Contact Name	170 – 199	30 Characters	Name of contact at group level that may receive access to their online reports. Do not provide vendor information. Vendors will not have access to private results. This field is required.

Jacquelene S. Hamer-McGhee, DNP, MSA, RN

Group Contact Phone	200 – 209	XXXXXX XXXX	10-digit phone number of group contact. *(do not include spaces or dashes.)*
Group Contact Email	210 – 239	30 Characters	Email address of contact at group level that may receive access to their CAHPS Database reports. This field is required.

Visit Survey Adult 2.0

Practice Site File Layout
Visit Survey Adult 2.0

Practice Site data file must be in ascii/flat format.
The file must contain one record for each Practice Site that administered the survey.
Practice Site and/or Group ID must match IDs in Sample and Group data files.
The data file must conform to the layout specifications below.

Variable Description	Field Position	Value Labels	Details/Comments
Practice Site ID	1-10	10 characters	Unique ID used to match the records in this Practice Site data file to the Sample Level data file & Group data file
Group ID	11-20	10 characters	Unique ID used to match the records in this Practice Site data file to the Sample Level & Group data file
Practice Site Name	21-70	50 characters	Name of the practice site used at the reporting level. Use unique names to help distinguish entities. This is the name that will appear in
Street	71-100	30	
Street	101-130	30	Floor or Suite

Jacquelene S. Hamer-McGhee, DNP, MSA, RN

City	131-160	30	
State	161-162	2	2-character State
Zip Code	163-167	XXXXX	5-digit zip code
Phone Number	168-177	XXXXXXXX XX	10-digit phone number. ***(do not include spaces or dashes.)***
Practice Ownership and Affiliation	178 – 179	01 = Provider(s) and/or Physician(s) 02 = Hospital or Health	Ownership or affiliation type that best describes this practice.
Patient Visits Per Week	180 – 184	XXXXX	5-digit number. What is the total number of patient visits in a typical week in this practice site
Providers Working Each Week	185 – 186	XX	2-digit number. What is the total number of providers (MDs, DOs, PAs, NPs, etc.) working in this practice site location during a typical week?
Sample Size	187 - 193	XXXXXXX	7-digit number. The sample size is the number of individuals drawn to receive a questionnaire for this practice site
Field Period Start	194 - 201	Mmddyyyy	8-digit date field. Date the survey fielding
Field Period End	202 - 209	Mmddyyyy	8-digit date field. Date the survey fielding

Visit Survey Adult 2.0

Variable Description	Field Position	Value Labels	Details/Comments
Response Rate	210 – 217	X.XXXX XX	8 spaces total, 6 decimal places. The response rate is the total number of completed returned questionnaires divided by the total number of respondents selected minus deceased and ineligible. For example, if 1,000 sampled patients yield 300 completed surveys minus 10 ineligible patients, the expected
Practice Contact Name	218 – 247	30 Characters	Name of contact at practice site that may receive access to their online report. Do not provide vendor information. Vendors will not have access to private
Practice Contact Phone	248 – 257	XXXXXX XXXX	10-digit phone number of practice contact. *(do not include spaces or dashes.)*
Practice Contact Email	258 – 287	30 Characters	Email address of contact at practice level that may receive access to their CAHPS Database reports

Sample File Layout

Visit Survey Adult 2.0

- Sample data file must be in ascii/flat format.
- The file must contain one record for each member in the sample.
- Practice Site and/or Group ID must match IDs in Practice Site and Group data files.
- The data file must conform to the layout specifications below.

Jacquelene S. Hamer-McGhee, DNP, MSA, RN

Variable	Field Position	Value	Details/Comments
Survey Type	1-2	33 = Visit Survey Adult 2.0	Indicates which instrument was used to administer the survey. **12-Month 4 Point Scale Instrument** 15 = 12-month Survey Adult 2.0 16 = 12-month PCMH Survey 2.0 (4pt) 17 = 12-month Survey Child 2.0 18 = 12-month PCMH Survey 2.0 (4pt) **Visit Instrument** 33 = Visit Survey Adult 2.0
Unique Record ID	3-12	10 characte	Unique ID for each record in the Sample
Practice Site ID	13-22	10 characte rs	Used to match the records in this Sample Level data file to the Practice Site data file
Group ID	23-32	10 characte rs	Used to match the records in this Sample Level data file to the Practice Site data file.
Provider NPI or ID	33-42	10	National Provider Identifier or a Unique ID for each Provider. Resident doctors can be submitted using Provider ID followed by 7 alphanumeric characters (i.e. res9A64944).
Provider First Name	43-62	20 characte	
Provider Last Name	63-82	20 characte	
Provider Specialty	83-85	001 = Allergy/l 003 = 004 = 005 = Dermato logy 006 = Diagnost 010 = 011 = 012 =	What **one** specialty category best describes **NEW:** Other health care professional specialty fields have been added to the list starting at value 101

Jacquelene S. Hamer-McGhee, DNP, MSA, RN

013 =
014 =
015 =
016 =
017 =
018 =
019 =
020 =
021 =
022 =
023 =
024 =

Visit Survey Adult 2.0

Variable	Field Position	Value Labels	Details/Comme
		025 = Pathology	
		026 = Pediatrics	
		027 = Physical	
		028 = Psychiatry	
		029 = Public	
		030 = Pulmonary	
		031 = Radiology	
		032 =	
		033 = Surgery	
		034 = Urology	
		035 = Vascular	
		036 = Internal	
		101 =	
		102 = Audiologist	
		103 = Certified	
		104 = Certified Anesthetist	
		105 = Clinical	
		106 = Clinical	
		107 = Clinical	
		108 = Nurse	
		109 =	
		110 = Physical	
		111 = Physician	
		112 = Registered Professional	
		113 = Speech-	
		998 = Other	
		999 = Missing	
Provider Gender	86	1 = Male	
		2 = Female	

Jacquelene S. Hamer-McGhee, DNP, MSA, RN

		9 = Missing	
Date of Last	87-94	Mmddyyyy 99999999 = Missing	8-digit date field **(do not include dashes or slashes)**
Survey Disposition Code	95-96	11 = Mail Complete 12 = Phone 14 = Web/Internet 15 = On Site 16 = Other 21 = Mail Partial 22 = Phone Partial 23 = IVR Partial 24 = Web/Internet 25 = On Site 26 = Other Partial 31 = Deceased 32 = Survey	Disposition that best represents final disposition for this
	1	33 = Language 34 = Unable to 35 = Unable to contact – Bad phone number 36 = Ineligible; mentally or 37 = Refused to complete survey 38 = Did not respond after maximum attempts	* On Site Complete = Survey completed at the Provider office Survey and Reporting Kit documents for additional
Survey	97-104	Mmddyyyy 99999999 = Missing	8-digit date field **(do not include dashes or slashes)**

Jacquelene S. Hamer-McGhee, DNP, MSA, RN

Variable	Field Position	Val	Details/Comme
Survey Complete Round	105-106	01 = 1st survey completed or 04 = 4th 05 = 5th survey completed or returned 06 = 6th survey	Indicates which mail, phone, web or IVR attempt If completed or returned survey after 6th attempt, indicate survey round (01 – 99 are ~~acceptable values~~
Survey Language	107	1 = English 2 = Spanish 3 = O	Other/Not applicable (use Disposition Code NOT equal to 11 – 26)
Patient Birth Year	108-111	Yyyy 9999 = Missing	Patient's year of birth Submission fails if all data are blank
Patient Gender	112	1 = Male 2 = Female 9 = Missing	
Patient zip code	113-117	xxxxx 99999 =	5-digit zip code
Q1. Our records show that you got care from the	118	1 = Yes 2 = No 8 = Multiple mark	
Q2. Is this the provider you usually see if you need a check-up, want advice about	119	1 = Yes 2 = No 7 = Appropriately skipped	
Q3. How long have you been going to this	120	1 = Less than 6 months 2 = At least 3 = At least 1 4 = At least 3 5 = 5 years or 7 = 8 = Multiple 9 = Missing	

Jacquelene S. Hamer-McGhee, DNP, MSA, RN

Q4.	In the last 12 months, how many times, did you visit	121-122	1 = None 2 = 1 time 3 = 2 4 = 3 5 = 4 6 = 5 to 9 7 = 10 or 77 = 88 = Multiple 99 = Missing
Q5.	In the last 12 months, did you phone this provider's office to get an appointment for	123	1 = Yes 2 = No 7 = Appropriately skipped 8 = Multiple

Visit Survey Adult 2.0

	Variable	Field Positio	Va	Details/Com
Q6.	In the last 12 when you provider's appointment needed right often did you appointme nt as soon	124	1 = Never 2 = 3 = Usually 4 = Always 7 = 8 = Multiple 9 = Missing	
Q7.	In the last 12 you make any appointments up or routine this provider?	125	1 = Yes 2 = No 7 = 8 = Multiple 9 = Missing	
Q8.	In the last 12 when you appointment up or routine this provider, did you get an appointme nt as soon	126	1 = Never 2 = 3 = Usually 4 = Always 7 = 8 = Multiple 9 = Missing	
Q9.	In the last 12 you phone office with a question	127	1 = Yes 2 = No 7 = 8 = Multiple	

Jacquelene S. Hamer-McGhee, DNP, MSA, RN

Q1	office hours? In the last 12 when you provider's regular office often did you answer to question that	128	9 = Missing 1 = Never 2 = 3 = Usually 4 = Always 7 = 8 = Multiple 9 = Missing
Q1	In the last 12 you phone office with a question after office hours?	129	1 = Yes 2 = No 7 = 8 = Multiple 9 = Missing
Q1	In the last 12 when you provider's regular office often did you answer to question as soon as you	130	1 = Never 2 = 3 = Usually 4 = Always 7 = 8 = Multiple 9 = Missing
Q1	Wait time spent in the and exam last 12 did you see within 15 appointment	131	1 = Never 2 = 3 = Usually 4 = Always 7 = 8 = Multiple 9 = Missing

Appendix D

Visit Survey Adult 2.0

Variable	Field Positio	Value	Details/Com
Q14. How since your most visit with this	132	1 = Less than 1 2 = At least 1 months 3 = At least 3 months but less 4 = At least 6 12 months 5 = 12 months or 7 = Appropriately 8 = Multiple mark	

Jacquelene S. Hamer-McGhee, DNP, MSA, RN

		9 = Missing
Q15. Wait time spent in the waiting and exam room. your most recent you see this provider within 15 minutes of your	133	1 = Yes 2 = No 7 = Appropriately 8 = Multiple Mark 9 = Missing
Q16. During visit, did this explain things in a that was easy to understand?	134	1 = Yes, definitely 2 = Yes, 3 = No 7 = Appropriately 8 = Multiple Mark 9 = Missing
Q17. During visit, did this listen carefully to	135	1 = Yes, definitely 2 = Yes, 3 = No 7 = Appropriately 8 = Multiple Mark 9 = Missing
Q18. During visit, did you talk provider about any questions or	136	1 = Yes 2 = No 7 = Appropriately 8 = Multiple Mark 9 = Missing
Q19. During visit, did this you easy to information about health questions or concerns?	137	1 = Yes, definitely 2 = Yes, 3 = No 7 = Appropriately 8 = Multiple Mark 9 = Missing
Q20. During visit, did this seem to know the important about your medical history?	138	1 = Yes, definitely 2 = Yes, 3 = No 7 = Appropriately 8 = Multiple Mark 9 = Missing
Q21. During visit, did this show respect for had to say?	139	1 = Yes, definitely 2 = Yes, 3 = No 7 = Appropriately 8 = Multiple Mark 9 = Missing
Q22. During visit, did this spend enough time you?	140	1 = Yes, definitely 2 = Yes, 3 = No 7 = Appropriately 8 = Multiple Mark

9 = Missing

Visit Survey Adult 2.0

Variable Description	Field Position	Value	Details/Co
Q23. During your most recent visit, did this provider order a	141	1 = Yes 2 = No 7 = Appropriately 9 = Missing	
Q24. Did someone from this provider's office	142	1 = Yes 2 = No 7 = 8 = Multiple 9 = Missing	
Q25. Using any number from 0 to 10, where 0 is the worst provider possible and 10 is the best provider possible, what	143-144	00 = 0 Worst provider possible 01 = 1 02 = 2 03 = 3 04 = 4 07 = 7 08 = 8 09 = 9 10 = 10 Best 77 = 88 = Multiple 99 = Missing	99 = Missing
Q26. Would you recommend this provider's office to	145	1 = Yes, definitely 2 = Yes, 7 = 8 = Multiple 9 = Missing	
Q27. During your most recent visit, were clerks and receptionists at this provider's office as helpful as you	146	1 = Yes, definitely 2 = Yes, somewhat 3 = No 7 =	

Jacquelene S. Hamer-McGhee, DNP, MSA, RN

Variable	Field Position	Value	Details/Comm
Q28. During your most recent visit, did clerks and receptionists at this provider's office treat you with	147	1 = Yes, definitely 2 = Yes, somewhat 3 = No 7 =	
Q29. In general, how rate your overall	148	1 = Excellent 2 = Very good 3 = Good 4 = Fair 5 = Poor 8 = Multiple 9 = Missing	Submission fails if are blank for this
Q30. In general, how would you rate your overall	149	1 = Excellent 2 = Very good 3 = Good 4 = Fair 5 = Poor 8 = Multiple 9 = Missing	

Visit Survey Adult 2.0

Variable	Field Position	Value	Details/Comm
Q31. What is your age?	150	1 = 18 to 24 2 = 25 to 34 3 = 35 to 44 4 = 45 to 54 5 = 55 to 64 6 = 65 to 74 7 = 75 or older 8 = Multiple Mark 9 = Missing	Submission fails if all data are blank for this field **AND** Patient Birth
Q32. Are you	151	1 = Male 2 = Female 8 = Multiple mark 9 = Missing	
Q33. What is the or level of school that you have	152	1 = 8th grade or 2 = Some high school, but did not 3 = High school 4 = Some college	Submission fails if **ALL** are blank for this field.

Jacquelene S. Hamer-McGhee, DNP, MSA, RN

		5 = 4-year college
		6 = More than 4-
		8 = Multiple Mark
		9 = Missing
Q34. Are you of Latino origin or	153	1 = Yes, Hispanic
		2 = No, not
		8 = Multiple Mark
		9 = Missing
Q35a. What is your race? Mark one or more.	154	0 = No.
Q35b. What is your race? Mark one or more.	155	0 = No
American		
Q35c. What is your race? Mark one or more.	156	0 = No
Q35d. What is your race? Mark one or more.	157	0 = No
Other Pacific What is your race? Mark one or more.	158	0 = No
○ Americ Alaska Native Q35f. What is your race? Mark one or more.	159	0 = No
Q36. Did someone help	160	1 = Yes
		2 = No
		8 = Multiple mark
		9 = Missing

Visit Survey Adult 2.0

Variable Description	Field Position	Value Labels	Details/Comments
Q37a. How did that vou? Mark one or ○ Read the questions to	161	0 = Not Selected 1 = Selected 7 = Appropriately skipped	
Q37b. How did that vou? Mark one or ○ Wrote down the answers I	162	0 = Not Selected 1 = Selected 7 = Appropriately skipped	
Q37c. How did that vou? Mark one or ○ Answered the questions for me	163	0 = Not Selected 1 = Selected 7 = Appropriately skipped	
Q37d. How did that vou? Mark one or ○ Translate d the questions into my language	164	0 = Not Selected 1 = Selected 7 = Appropriately skipped	
Q37e. How did that vou? Mark one or ○ Helped in some other way	165	0 = Not Selected 1 = Selected 7 = Appropriately skipped	

About the Author

Jacquelene S. Hamer-McGhee possesses more than three decades of experience in clinical and healthcare operations. In roles as Chief Patient Experience Officer, Deputy Chief of Clinical Informatics and Tele-Health Services, she has focused on the patient and family healthcare experience and healthcare informatics, while utilizing her skills in quality and process improvement, strategic management, and large-scale change management. In addition, as a clinical registered nurse and healthcare administrator, Dr. Hamer-McGhee has focused her work on the patient/family experience, care delivery systems, and evidence-based practice. She earned her Doctor of Nursing Practice degree from American Sentinel University and a Master of Science in Information Resource Management from Central Michigan University. She is a servant leader in her professional career as well as her personal life. Jacquelene serves as a small group leader for both an international bible study program and young adults in her home church. Her interests include addressing healthcare disparities, healthcare literacy and holistic wellness.

Jacquelene S. Hamer-McGhee, DNP, MSA, RN

www.ingramcontent.com/pod-product-compliance
Lightning Source LLC
Chambersburg PA
CBHW020324290526
45785CB00007B/2913